REFLECTIONS

OF A FORMER

FATTY

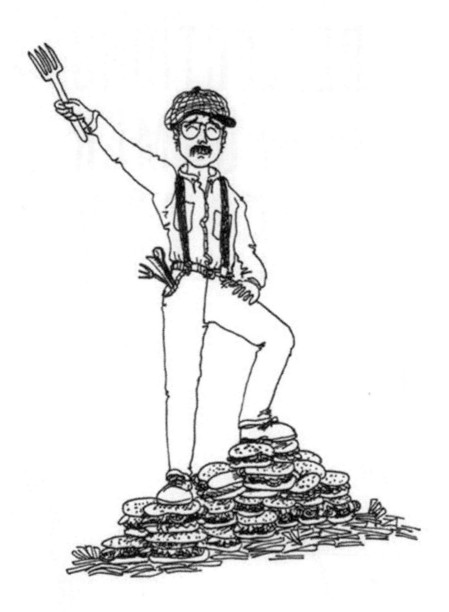

REFLECTIONS OF A FORMER FATTY

HOW TO WIN THE WAR AGAINST WEIGHT ONCE AND FOR ALL

THOM SLAGLE

ISBN: 979-8-89031-700-1 (sc)
ISBN: 979-8-89031-701-8 (hc)
ISBN: 979-8-89031-702-5 (e)
Library of Congress Control Number: 2013907263

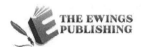
THE EWINGS
PUBLISHING

One Galleria Blvd., Suite 1900, Metairie, LA 70001
(504) 702-6708

For my sweet Elizabeth.

It's been well worth the wait.

I'm thin but fun.

—Woody Allen

In memory of

Herman H. Hepner, MD
(1927–1992)

Dr. Herman Hepner never had any doubts about his career choice, following his mother, father, grandfather, and two uncles into the field of medicine. For thirty-seven years, he was a dedicated physician in the same small Midwestern community that welcomed him in 1953. Dr. Hepner was well known for his gentle bedside manner and the compassion he displayed in his approach to practicing medicine. He passed away in November 1992 from cancer of the bone marrow, from which he suffered for a year and a half. Dr. Hepner is remembered by family, friends, and colleagues as a quiet, devoted family man.

Dr. Herman Hepner saved my life.

TABLE OF CONTENTS

ILLUSTRATIONS

FIGURES

ACKNOWLEDGMENTS

There are so many people to thank for their efforts in bringing this book to print. First and foremost, I would like to acknowledge the wonderful contribution of Beth W. Reasoner, whose illustrations give extraordinary life to ordinary and mere words. An enormous thank-you also to Julia Robinson, PhD, who dissected the approaches and methodologies and endorsed and supported the behavioral techniques employed within these pages. A special thank-you goes to Marian Hepner; without her blessings and consent this book would not have been possible.

I would especially like to acknowledge the late Herman Hepner, MD, whose wisdom, inspiration, and advice guided the creation of the weight-loss approach described in this book. Without his influence and counsel, this book could not have been written.

In the course of attempting to lose weight, I read a number of books on dieting and making better eating and lifestyle choices. Among those were *The Doctor's Quick Weight Loss Diet* by Dr. Irwin Maxwell Stillman, commonly known as the Stillman Diet, which was published in 1967, as well as several others that appeared on the weight-loss landscape in later years, such as the 1972 *Diet Revolution* by Dr. Robert Atkins and much later, his *Dr. Atkins New Revolution Diet*, both of which promoted a low-carbohydrate diet plan. I even tried the so-called diet shakes that followed the advent of Knudsen Creamery Company's *Diet 225* drinks that, over time, flooded the market. Each of these, in its own right, served a very useful purpose in the weight-loss wars. I deeply appreciate the wisdom and insight each book provided.

To the countless others who directly or indirectly influenced, encouraged, and otherwise championed my endeavors to win the Battle of the Bulge, I extend my heartfelt gratitude.

And to my wonderful Elizabeth, I thank you for your sage advice, honest critique, and support regarding this manuscript. Most importantly, I thank you for your boundless love. You truly are the most important person in my life, and you make me a far better person than I ever thought possible.

INTRODUCTION

FOOD FOR THOUGHT

Someone once said that the best things in life come in small packages. There is a great deal of truth to that statement. So I bought into it. That is one reason why this book is not as massive as many of the other books dealing with similar topics. Of course, there are other reasons for its lack of girth, beginning with the psychological factor. It just made sense that a manuscript exhorting a weight-loss program should be relatively *thin*. Then there's the simple reason that I had said all I had wanted to say, and the length of this book is exactly how long it took me to say it.

The weight-loss approach chronicled within these pages is not a diet program. Diets require the participant to give up certain great-tasting foods. The effects of successful diets are magnified through increased energy and exercise, yet many overlook certain "issues" that plague people who give these diets a try. Why? Well, for one, I've always suspected that virtually all diets were created by skinny guys in white lab coats who really didn't have a clue as to the inherent problems we People of Excessive Weight must constantly confront. If you've read some of these diet books, you probably know what I mean. Most of us are not really keen on that whole giving-up-good-tasting-food thing; many of us are not disciplined enough to want to weigh or measure portions. We often lack stamina or the wherewithal to stick with any diet that doesn't produce quick results. Then there's this thing called willpower, and so many of us have no clue what it actually is. Many of our problems are rooted in the *psychology* of weight loss.

That's why this approach was created. Unlike many of the diet books of the era, it doesn't make you give up this or that kind of food. You won't have to measure or weigh portions—at least not in a traditional sense. It sets the bar far lower. Really low, actually.

This plan was not developed in a laboratory in a spooky, remote castle, but rather in the context of real life. It was created by a fat person who was—excuse the pun—fed up with being fat and out of shape and thoroughly frustrated by his inability to lose weight by conventional means. With the help of his trusted family physician, this successful plan for losing weight was developed through a process of trial and error. There were various obstacles and hurdles that had to be dealt with at every turn. When something didn't work, it was analyzed and analyzed again to determine why it didn't work. Then adjustments were made in the methodology to compensate for it. And it worked like a charm. How do I know? I was that fat person.

When I first began this weight-loss saga some forty years ago, I had no idea whether this cockamamie scheme of mine would work during the course of three or four days, let alone whether it would be effective for a decade or two. I just knew that I had to do something radical, or chances were ... well, let's just say I didn't see a very bright future on the horizon.

The methods employed in this program to lose weight—and keep it off—were based on very basic common sense. I went with my instincts, relying solely on what I believed would work for me. It was all predicated on what my family doctor—who knew me medically better than anyone else—suggested and recommended.

Very simply, this program taught me how to develop that ever-elusive concept called *willpower*. How was that accomplished? By learning to *moderate* my food portions gradually, over time. I developed the *mental fortitude* it takes to say "enough is enough" when it really is enough. It really is quite easy.

I did not have to sacrifice a single, solitary food to enjoy the benefits of my newfound willpower. I ate every food I loved—only I ate far less than I was accustomed to eating. But I still felt quite satisfied after every meal, and you can—and *will*—too.

Food for thought. *Bon appetit!*

PART ONE

REFLECTIONS OF A FORMER FATTY

CHAPTER ONE

THE WINDS OF WAR

I can tell you—as if you really need reminding—it's no fun being fat. I speak from experience. I can't remember a time when I wasn't, at the very least, incredibly chubby.

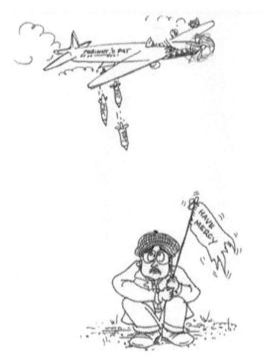

My life was spent constantly dodging the bombardment
of fat that seemed to just naturally fall from the sky.

My life was spent constantly dodging the bombardment of fat that seemed to just naturally fall from the sky—and attach itself to my waistline. I just didn't know how to avoid getting hit by it. Truth was, I didn't try really hard to get out of its way.

I'm pretty certain that no one really wants to be fat. I know I didn't actually ask anyone to make me fat. At least not that I can remember. Given their druthers, I think most guys would rather look more like Paul Newman—well, when he was alive at least—or George Clooney than Jabba the Hutt. I'd imagine women would prefer to have an alluring figure in the tradition of, say, an Elizabeth Taylor or Kate Winslet than one of those dancing hippos in *Fantasia*. Really, when was the last time you heard someone lament about not being *fat* enough to be a supermodel? Yeah, that's what I thought.

My love of eating was not the result of some deeply rooted psychological trauma. The reality was, I simply had an enormous appetite and ate all I wanted, whenever I wanted, to satisfy those tremendous pangs of hunger that called to me from within my ever-expanding stomach. It seems, though, that I had a selective hunger. I never craved—or seldom ate—anything that the food gods deemed healthy. No, I chose to munch on food that tasted great—and apparently was loaded with tons of sugar and calories.

After years of pretty much forsaking any remotely healthy food, I woke up one morning to an epiphany. It wasn't quite like having visions of sugarplums dancing in my head, but it was still pretty cool. As I was rocking back and forth to gain the momentum I needed to extricate myself from the comfort of my bed, I realized that my problem with weight—as with most everything else in my life—was due to one teeny-tiny flaw: I had absolutely no *willpower*. That was especially true when it came to eating. Because I lacked the willpower to stay away from the foods I loved, and I lacked the initiative and drive to get out and exercise, I was never going to be thin. Not even close to it.

How It Came to Pass That I Got Fat

Exactly how I arrived at the point of being overtly pudgy is difficult to say with any certainty. Naturally, I have theories, and I'm going to share those theories here and now.

Whereas some kids are born with a proverbial silver spoon in their mouths, I kinda figured out that I was delivered into this world with a *sugar* spoon in my mouth. How sweet is *that!* Just as those little silver-spooners didn't have to work to get rich, I learned from a very young age that I didn't have to work to get fat. While they just had to sit around, doing little more than watching their trust funds grow, I figured out pretty quickly that all I had to do was sit around and eat to watch my waistline grow. Those kids got rich. This kid got fat.

This being-born-with-a-sugar-spoon-in-my-mouth thing probably contributed significantly to my weight problems as I grew older and began making food choices for myself. I just couldn't stay away from any type of sweet dessert—even when there was no dessert to be found in the house. The cravings eventually drove me to take extreme measures at the oddest times to satisfy the urges.

It began simply enough by slipping into the kitchen under the cover of night and making cinnamon-and-sugar toast—oftentimes two, three, or even four slices. Okay, I confess that it wasn't unusual for me to enjoy this sumptuous snack even when dessert had been served at dinner.

By the time I was twelve, I could no longer stand and see my feet, for the size of my stomach. I can't recall exactly how much I weighed back then, but if I wasn't medically morbidly obese, I was certainly getting close. Still, my cravings for tasty, sugar-laden snacks were so profound that I "needed" to supplement the selection available at home with a greater variety. But to purchase these new delights, I needed money, so I sought gainful employment.

I scored a job at the local Dairy Queen, which was like this really huge *coup de maitre* for a fat kid. It was like being in hog heaven, so to speak.

The one really healthy thing that came from my DQ experience was that it introduced me to the importance of fruit in one's diet. I began eating strawberry sundaes, banana splits, even an occasional pineapple sundae for a taste of the exotic. I hadn't realized how good fruit tasted until then. So I kept expanding my foray into the world of yummy "fruit"—while not quite understanding why my waist was expanding at such an alarming rate.

I had also ventured off to middle school, where I got my first exposure to warm lunches and a "balanced" school meal. This balance included selections from the five basic food groups: grains and starch; fruit and vegetables; milk and dairy; meat, fish, and poultry; and, my personal favorite, fats and sugars. The portions were doled out into little sections of plastic trays. I tried these lunches for a while but was always left wanting—craving, even—more. There just wasn't enough of the good-tasting foods that I longed for. "Balanced," my fat fanny!

Figure 1.
Five Basic Food Groups

The USDA has identified five basic food groups. A healthy diet consists of food from all those groups in correct portions to provide energy and growth to the human body.

Grains and Starch	Fruits and Vegetables	Milk and Dairy	Meat, Fish, and Poultry	Fats and Sugars
• Bread, pasta, potatoes, rice, noodles, cereal • Food belonging to this group should be the main part of every meal • These foods are the main source of fiber and vitamin B • High fiber variety is suggested	• Excellent source of natural vitamins, minerals, fibers • Have low fat and less calories • Regular diet should include minimum of 5 portions of fruit and vegetable servings	• Milk, cheese, yogurt • Rich source of protein, vitamins, calcium, and minerals • Required servings: 3 per day • Should prefer lowfat versions to avoid saturated fat	• Major source of iron and vitamin B12 • In red meat, visible fats should be cut and discarded; choose leaner portions • Red meat should be eaten once a week • Fish should be eaten twice a week • Lentils, nuts, beans, and peas are good, and a regular diet should include at least 2 portions every day	• Butter, cream, ice cream, cakes, cooking oils, low-fat spreads, mayo, margarine, sugary drinks, salad dressings, biscuits, chocolate, sweets, pastries • These types of foods should be avoided because they are high in fat and calories • Better options are low sugar or sugar-free sweets and snacks

Source: adipexpower.com; US Department of Agriculture.

I just knew that I had to do something to supplement this whole "balanced diet" thing. Little did I know that it was waiting for me just beyond the school grounds.

What I discovered was a quaint neighborhood grocery store just down the block from the school, where I could pick out a couple of handfuls of candy. This, by my way of thinking, was all the "balance" I needed in my diet. Shoot, I would even stop at that store frequently on my way home from school in the afternoon. I justified these after-school delights because I had a long walk home and needed the quick boost in energy to get there. We didn't have energy drinks back when I was a kid. Strangely, despite my balanced meals and plenty of exercise I got from walking, my waist just kept getting bigger and bigger.

After I got my driver's license, the extreme measures reached a whole new level. When those cravings attacked me in the middle of the night, I no longer had to resort to what was available to me in house. Oh, no. I could simply hop in the car, drive a mile or so west, and feast on all kinds of really yummy baked goods at the local all-night truck stop. The restaurant always featured great pies, cakes, even donuts virtually 24/7. How could I resist? Of course, I never did—which is one theory as to why I probably got fat.

Looking back on my childhood, there were other reasons why I probably got really, really pudgy. To begin with, my mom used to prepare a dinner almost every night that consisted of something like nine or twelve courses. I was always astounded at how huge the meals were. Being the polite child that I was, I would make sure that I ate each course. It was only years and several pounds later that I learned my mom never served that many courses in actuality. It turns out that I was simply helping myself to multiple servings of just the main course—sometimes three or four helpings at a sitting. But I always had room for dessert, because that's how I rolled—very nearly literally.

In my defense, though, I did once attempt to eat less while still a child. I was actually losing weight to the point that I was just kind of chubby, rather than enormous. Heck, I had actually begun wearing "husky" clothes instead of "fat" ones. Then we took a family vacation to see my maternal grandparents. That turned out to be a big, um, fat mistake, any way you looked at it.

Not only did my grandmother prepare a lavish spread for every meal, but there were always great-smelling—and -tasting—desserts calling my name from the kitchen. Constantly.

Despite these temptations, however, I was bound and determined to stick to my newfound weight-loss plan at any cost. So I resisted—to the best of my youthful ability. But here's the problem: my grandmother was practically deaf, so when I would shout something like, "That's enough," she apparently thought I was saying, "More stuff," and filled my plate with more helpings of everything. Being the polite child I was, I would make sure I ate everything on my plate—two, three, four times. A boy can only protest so often, you know. I certainly did not want to cross my grandmother, a very stern, foreboding sort, who ruled the household with an iron fist and a look that could kill a grown man at forty paces.

Heck, she was so scary that my soft-spoken, gentle grandfather would hide from her in his basement retreat. He always said he had something to do down there, but I suspect it was to keep her from piercing him with *that* look. Can't say as I blamed him. That is another theory as to why I probably got fat.

Perhaps most significant was the theory that I got fat as a public service. During my formative years, my future girth was influenced heavily—again, no pun intended—by a song I heard on a record album my parents had. Against a backdrop of "America the Beautiful," the singer explained how he had gotten fat because his mother would tell him to clean his plate "because children were starving in Europe." Interestingly, my mother used to tell me the exact same thing. Thinking it would keep the children in Europe from going hungry, the singer would clean his plate four, five, even six times a day. But alas, the children kept starving, and he got fat. Because my mother framed it the way she did, I just thought it was a small way—even my duty—in which I could help those poor, hungry kids in Europe. So I cleaned my plate at least that many times a day. But, alas and alack, children kept starving, and *I* got fat!

As a final exhortation that it was not in vain that he got fat, the singer suggested that it was every normal person's patriotic duty whenever they saw a fat person to say—in a loud, yet reverential voice—to that fat person, "Hail to thee, fat person! You kept us out of war!" I just felt so … I don't know, humble and peacefully American, doing what I did.

How It Came to Pass That I Got Thin

There comes a time when everyone seems to take stock in their lives. They look at the things they failed to accomplish and those they succeeded in achieving. I was no different—well, I *was* different, but not regarding this taking-stock-in-my-life thing. The main difference was that I could never come up with any accomplishments or achievements, so I made the decision to evaluate only those glaring failures in my life and leave it at that. After completing one such reflection, I arrived at what I thought was an interesting observation. When most people carry around the weight of the world, it's usually on their shoulders. For me, it was quite apparent that I had—for some strange and unknown reason—chosen to carry the weight of the world attached firmly to my waist. And no matter what, it refused to let go.

I often looked at diets as being this never-ending journey where my feet were moving and the scenery was changing, but I just never seemed to get anywhere. It was as if I was caught up in a surreal trap in which the backdrop was manipulated to create the illusion that I was moving and making progress. It was a bit like one of those old-fashioned shooting galleries at a carnival, where the objects just kept moving back and forth before the shooter's eyes, with no way to escape. I figured it out eventually and jumped *off* the bandwagon of false promises and deceit.

That realization pushed me to develop a plan that I could follow without failing, because I became frustrated with the whole idea. So, that's what I did—developed a plan, I mean, not the got-frustrated-with-the-whole-idea thing. Although there was that, of course.

The plan I came up with takes into account the natural struggles that have prevented success for so many who have taken the walk down the primrose path to what they anticipated would be a great and successful reduction in weight. It conveniently cuts through the creeping, clinging vines of frustration that cause us to falter and fall and consequently bruise our gentle yet fragile psyches as we take each step toward the promised land of weight loss.

I have always considered myself to be a rather passive, gentle kind of guy. I certainly am not the type to go fight someone or some*thing*— especially if there were other options available, like running in the opposite direction as fast as my chubby little legs could trundle. So I was more than a little surprised by what happened to me.

At the time I finally made the decision to do something about my weight, I was struggling with simple daily tasks. I couldn't even bend over to tie my shoelaces without gasping for breath. That's how heavy I had gotten.

I had to prepare myself mentally for the undertaking that lay ahead. I had to *want* to lose weight, not just do it for the sake of doing it. I *needed* to understand that if I continued on the path I was traveling, I was going to die before my time. It really was that serious.

While I am not hawkish or a warmonger by any stretch of the imagination, I decided that the only way to finally lose weight was to declare war on all things that challenged my attempts to accomplish that. It's not as if I went to the local army surplus store and bought a bunch of paramilitary gear. Nor did I break into an armory somewhere and borrow all kinds of implements of destruction. It wasn't going to be that kind of war. No, I decided to declare a *mental* war on weight instead. It was much less physically exhausting that way and less likely to be fatal—which was more than just a small concern to me. I mean, really. If I had *actually* gone to war and been fatally wounded, it would've made writing this book very, very difficult.

I equate the effort to lose weight with fighting a war. It's not just a physical endeavor. So much of losing weight is *psychological.* Soldiers fighting wars on any front have to make life-and-death decisions in the face of the enemy. Oftentimes, those of us who battle the war with weight must be as decisive with the choices we have to make. One could argue that losing weight is a serious proposition when it comes to potentially saving a life. I know that was the case with me.

I didn't have any real practical experience in waging war, although I conducted any number of combat missions in the war-ravaged vacant lot in the neighborhood of my youth. But it didn't stop there. When the weather was too miserable to be outside fighting wars, I would break out the Battleground play set that I got for Christmas one year, and I never lost a single battle. So I learned a thing or two about fighting battles in the comfort of my home as well. This was important, by my way of thinking, because most of this war on weight was going to be fought at home. In any event, I may not have the expertise of, say, a general, but I thought I'd reached the level of a colonel.

So it was that I put down my knife, fork, and spoon, and I picked up a pen and pad of paper. Rather than field maps containing the position of enemy troops, I studied book after book containing the positions of several diet programs. Rather than carrying a flask of courage to calm my nerves on the battlefield, I brought along a cocktail of intuition and determination to carry me through the battle I was about to wage. Before I marched off to the battleground, I diligently prepared a plan of attack to fight my war on weight. The winds of war were not just blowing, they were blowing with gale force.

What follows is a true story.

CHAPTER TWO

WHISPERS OF INSURGENCY

After years of submitting to a variety of diets, so-called healthy-living schemes, and what I can only describe as ritualistic hogwash, I was convinced that I was destined to remain for life a Person of Excessive Weight. Not that I wanted to be, mind you. Quite honestly, I thought about food practically all the time. It was simply that I loved to eat and hated to exercise—an extremely dangerous combination even by most devil-may-care gluttonous standards.

These "healthy-lifestyle programs" promised that they would make me lean and fit. That certainly was all well and good and made for a great read. I was all gung-ho to jump into this new wave of fitness and health with all my heart and soul, except for one little matter. On closer examination, I discovered that the promise of a very svelte me came with an enormous price tag, one that went well beyond the financial. This whole-new-me thing would only work if I was willing and able to cut out foods that I loved and cherished more than life itself. Oh, and then these programs seemed to herald a regimen of rigorous exercise in order for them to make me thin. Nice try.

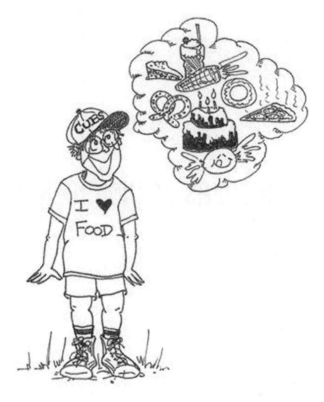

But quite honestly, I thought about food practically all the time.

Nevertheless, I was a trouper. I think I tried to follow every diet plan that was published from the late '60s on. I actually remember lasting about three days on one of them without cheating. I considered that a moral—if not somewhat empty—victory. The others were so much worse, if you can believe it. Just reading about what was expected of me made me grab as many cookies and donuts as my chubby little fingers could get ahold of and shove in my mouth. Staying on a diet and losing weight were just way too much work, as far as I could tell. Basically, I was fat and lazy and easily discouraged by all the work involved with losing weight.

Then in late 1970, certain unforeseeable events happened that changed my attitude about how I wanted to live and, consequently, altered my way of thinking about this being-fat thing. Those events breathed life into a program of smarter eating and a healthier lifestyle—without sacrifice—that has proven successful for me, a naturally lazy, lethargic kind of guy who was prone to being overweight but not necessarily liking it.

I refer to the program as being a common-sense approach to changing your lifestyle because it *is* a common-sense approach to changing your lifestyle. The whole program is predicated on just that: common sense. The only expert I consulted was my family physician, mostly as a matter of prudence, rather than to seek out his advice. In retrospect, however, his wisdom and the unique manner in which he dealt with me were incredibly insightful, influential, and inspirational—and directly responsible for my ultimate success in losing weight.

In developing this approach, I analyzed the reasons why I could not be true to other programs created by so-called experts and then made allowances for them. For example, I taught myself the elusive concept known as willpower by moderating my consumption over a period of time. I designed the approach to reduce my excess weight gradually. I believed that not only is it healthier to lose weight a little at a time, but the weight is more inclined to stay off if it is lost slowly. Besides, that was one thing my family doctor recommended, so it made sense to me. It was a matter of trial and error—a few subtle adjustments being made from time to time but with no concessions to speak of. I didn't really weigh or measure the food I was eating, nor did I give up any of the great-tasting foods I was very fond of.

What began merely as a self-designed personal weight-loss program ultimately became a new lifestyle, even though I hadn't planned it that way. The fact of the matter is, this newfangled approach was developed by a person who has continuously waged a battle of the bulge—not by people who profess to know what is best for people like you and me.

By golly, the approach worked for me, and it has been successful for more than four decades. There have been lapses here and there, but each of them was beaten once I realized how tightly my clothes were fitting—or when some other obnoxious sign reared its ugly head. For instance, when I'd pass a full-length mirror and catch a glimpse of my reflection out of the corner of my eye. It was ghastly, simply ghastly.

Obviously, there are no guarantees that you will succeed in losing weight on this plan. But as you read this book, you will realize that the concepts are radically different than any other plan you've ever read or heard about. You may agree that it could actually work for you. It simply makes sense.

If there's one thing I learned from reading and analyzing all these diet plans, it's that they just assumed a person could follow their instructions and do all the things each plan expected them to do, whether it was giving up certain foods or measuring stuff or exercising or whatever. For many, losing weight goes beyond being a simple challenge.

But there wasn't a diet on the market that seemed to encourage my efforts. That was the real problem. I couldn't envision being slender when there was no end to the dieting in sight. That was one major issue addressed with this approach.

I also knew that I could not measure out helpings of food—certainly not immediately. I didn't have the wherewithal to go from eating whatever, whenever—and as much as I wanted—without having extreme hunger pangs coaxing me to eat and eat and eat to my heart's content. So that issue was addressed as well.

Eventually, I found the ideal method by which to develop willpower while keeping an "eye on the prize," as it were. I decided to declare war on my weight by establishing a systematic approach that attacked the very core of my weight problems.

While I didn't don any military gear or fight with the implements of destruction associated with going into a conventional battle, my fight was tactical and deliberate. The great thing is, the program brought me success where only failure and despair once existed. If I could do it, I am absolutely certain that *anyone* who suffers the same issues with losing weight can follow this plan and enjoy the sweet taste of victory. Literally.

So let's get to it, shall we? There's a war to be fought that we will finally win—the Battle of the Bulge!

CHAPTER THREE

A CALL TO ARMS

I was the stereotypical fat kid in the neighborhood. You know the type—the kid whose T-shirt was always so tight that the ridges of fat stuck out around his waist like he forgot to step out of the cute ducky-float thing after he got done swimming.

The point is that from my preteen years through my days as a teenager, the weight hung around my middle, silently announcing to the world that I was pretty much a sorry slob who had no concept of how to be healthy. No ifs, ands, or buts about it. Fat is fat and that is that.

For as long as I can remember, whenever sides were being chosen for games of sport or recreation, I was almost always the last person picked. The group of kids waited along the sidelines, eager to be given that verbal acknowledgment of acceptance by the "better" kids—the power-mongers of the playground, if you will—with a pointed finger and a simple, "I'll take you." I couldn't help but look around whenever that affirmation was directed at me—if only to see how many others were still lingering. More times than not, there weren't any.

It didn't matter that I was as good as or better than most of the others selected before me. All that counted to my classmates and friends was that I was overweight, and that meant—automatically—that everybody else *had* to be better. To them, I couldn't run as fast or maneuver as well; I couldn't shoot the basketball with as much accuracy or hit a baseball as far. In the minds of my playmates and peers, I was fat and just plain no good. Period. That's just how it was back when I was a kid—and pretty much how it is to this day, I'd imagine.

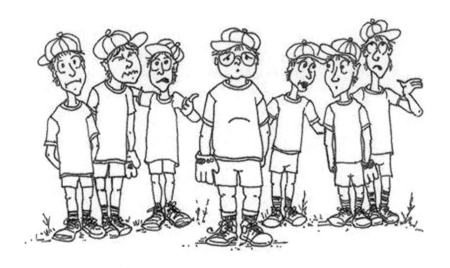

I was almost always the last person picked from
the group of kids along the sidelines.

Despite the taunting jeers of my classmates and the looks of disdain from complete strangers—slender people mostly, I might add—I was pretty much a happy kid. A cheerful disposition and disarming wit shielded me from the sting of criticism and were, despite my growing weight problem, magnets in attracting more than my share of acquaintances and friends.

My life was basically pretty serene and enjoyable. I just had a couple of minor little personality quirks: I loved to eat and hated to exercise. It didn't make me a bad person, mind you, despite what others would try to get me to believe with their relentless taunts. Actually, my life nowhere resembled a psychological shambles.

My love of eating was not the result of some deeply rooted psychological trauma that reared its ugly head. It didn't manifest itself in my need to devour the rest of the half-eaten chocolate layer cake or to help myself to seconds, thirds, and sometimes, fourths of nightly dinners. I came about it quite naturally.

As a matter of fact, I had a loving, nurturing childhood. I simply had a real weakness for all those wonderfully tantalizing baked goods and great-tasting dishes that were conjured up in the kitchen on a daily basis—each aroma my personal siren of temptation. So I don't put much substance in those psychological profiles and studies that suggest otherwise.

Overweight, out-of-shape people are not bad people, any more than slender, fit people are. In many cases, the problem isn't terribly complex at all. It's often as simple as having an enormous appetite and eating all you want to satisfy the mystical pangs of hunger that coax you from inside that ever-expanding stomach. Simple as that.

I avoided virtually all forms of known and accepted exercise and ignored the mild protestations of my parents, other relatives, and all my friends concerning my eating habits. I was just a normal kid who loved to eat. There was nothing really terribly ominous about it.

So what changed my mind, you may ask? In late 1970, I was nineteen years old, cocky and arrogant—and about fifty pounds overweight. At least if you believed those statistical charts that are published by so-called experts—no doubt, *thin* ones—who profess to know such things.

I was still a happy-go-lucky person, quick with a smile and a joke, and still eating what felt like twice my weight in food at each sitting. In other words, nothing much had changed to this point in my life. I was eating whatever I wanted, whenever I wanted. And exercise, to me, was having to hoist myself up from my easy chair in front of the television to grab another bag of cookies or make another sandwich. Or both.

The day before Thanksgiving that year, an event occurred that would have a profound and lasting effect on my family and me.

My father—always a picture of strength and health, by my way of thinking—suffered a heart attack. I might add that this happened while he was sitting in his easy chair in front of the television.

Although it was not a massive coronary, that did not diminish the fear and anxiety that ripped through my family's veil of contentment. A fine line separates life from death and, for the first time, my family was forced to examine just how fine and sharp a line it really is—up close and personal. For the first time in my life, I was truly frightened. My father was no longer strong and invincible. Now he was pale and weak and completely vulnerable. Quite frankly, it scared the hell out of me. If ever two people were cast from identical molds, it was my father and me. Suddenly, I was staring at the inevitability of death, lying motionless in a hospital bed with tubes and needles and monitors and nurses and doctors everywhere. Sure, it was my father lying there. But the image I saw was me.

I realized at that moment that unless I preferred death to life, I was going to have to do something dramatic about my devil-may-care approach to life and my expanding waistline. I was going to have to get myself in shape, no matter how I felt about the whole thing. I was going to have to whip myself into shape by—ugh—dieting. Yikes!

CHAPTER FOUR

DEPLOYING THE TROOPS

O f course, that epiphany begged the question, how was I going to accomplish this dieting thing? I mean, I was as lazy as a guy could be and still be considered ambulatory. And I did *love* to eat. So how could I possibly go about it with any hope at all of succeeding?

The plan was really quite simple. I went out and purchased—for a small fortune, I might add—virtually every book that had ever been written on the subject of dieting. You name it, I bought it.

Because I anticipated many battles with my fragile psyche during my self-declared war on weight, I also bought a library of self-help and self-realization books to better prepare myself to attack the powerful urge to do what I often did best in situations like these: simply to say "to hell with everything" and just go on doing what I did so well from the comfort of my easy chair in front of the television. My philosophy was, since I could no longer feed my stomach, the least I could do was feed my mind. I suppose it was a reasonable trade-off.

I spent the next few days holed up in my room, perusing my newly acquired library and jotting down notes of comparison and differences between each of the program offerings. All the while, I was shoveling mountains of junk food into my mouth like there was no tomorrow. Feed the mind, feed the stomach. Funny, how that works.

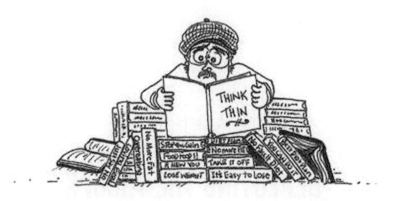

I went out and purchased every book that had ever
been written on the subject of dieting.

What I discovered from this research was that while each plan certainly seemed legitimate—even potentially beneficial—all of them were substantially flawed, at least from the perspective of those who love to eat. Here's why. Each diet plan that I reviewed practically forced me to fail at losing weight from the get-go. They made me work hard, weighing all those yucky veggies and stuff they essentially wanted to force-feed me and had me forsake the near and dear—namely, most of those glorious foods that set my taste buds aflutter with excitement and my tummy rumbling with gurgles of delight. That certainly was not gonna happen.

One point that each of these books made seemed very prudent: before you consider pursuing any weight-reduction plan—including the one you're reading about right now—consult your physician or a health-care professional. *It is absolutely imperative.* Enough said about that.

So after weeks of mental fatigue and utter frustration, and having failed in my efforts to follow any of the programs for more than three days or so, that's precisely what I did. I made an appointment and went to visit my family doctor.

Herman Hepner had been my family's physician for most of my nineteen years, so it's pretty safe to say that he knew me and each member of my family better than just about anyone, physiologically speaking. His bedside manner made you feel like you were the only patient he had, despite a waiting room that rivaled the population of Rhode Island at any given time. He was always careful to take the time to talk in depth about whatever medical issues his patients believed they had, and he always spoke candidly with each person he encountered. He was a man of great medical knowledge and infinite wisdom. To this day, I credit him for the success I achieved with this program.

It was his candor about dieting and his encouragement that convinced me to give weight loss one more shot. His guidance and understanding were paramount in the development of what was to become an approach to eating better and living a healthier life that actually worked for me.

As attending physician to my father, Dr. Hepner was of course already completely aware of his situation. We spoke briefly concerning my father's condition, and then I cut to the chase, explaining to him that I was concerned about my health—being so fat and out of shape—and wanted him to put me on a diet to save my life. Not that I had a flair for the dramatic or anything.

He nodded knowingly at everything I said, and for the longest time, he just sat there on his little black stool at his little white table, looking over what I imagined was the horror story that was my medical record. For a while, I thought he may have dozed off during some of the more boring parts, but then he'd give a "hmm" and flip the page. Once, I could've sworn that I heard a throaty chuckle—but I'm not entirely sure. There may even have been an audible gasp or two as well.

After several moments of contemplating the silent comedy of horrors that was my medical information, he turned to gaze intently at the acoustical ceiling tiles—in all likelihood using his laser vision to burn still more tiny holes into those squares—as he considered my request. Then his gaze moved from the ceiling tiles—apparently he was done boring more holes—and settled on me.

He paused briefly and then said point-blank, "I don't believe in diet plans. And even if I did, you wouldn't follow any of them." (I told you he was a man of infinite wisdom, didn't I?) Of course, the way he said it, so matter-of-factly, made my heart sink. I figured right then and there that I was just doomed to be fat and live a short, unfulfilled life as a result.

Hearing those few words left me feeling so despondent, so hopeless that I actually thought the unthinkable: it was time to find a different doctor. Despite his wisdom, despite his *savoir faire*, it was all I could do to keep from dropping to my knees, grabbing his pant leg, and begging and pleading for him to reconsider. Given the lack of any willpower in my life, I was surprised that I hadn't.

Instead I just sat there on the examination table, staring sadly at the drab walls, not knowing exactly what to think or do. The way I looked at it was, *heck, I would have felt better had he pulled out a loaded revolver, aimed it directly at my chest, and pulled the trigger.* By my way of thinking, I was gonna die before my time, one way or another. Just at that moment, though, a small miracle occurred.

He completely agreed with me about my need to lose weight or end up dead before my time. That being observed, the program was launched in a rather unceremonious manner. The first step was to conduct a cursory physical examination, which Dr. Hepner performed right there in his office. The exam consisted mostly of checking all my vital signs for any abnormalities. There were no serious ones, fortunately. Then, with a great sigh and a certain amount of trepidation, I stepped onto the gleaming white-black-and-silver Scales of Truth—(and injustice)—for the bane of a fat person's existence: the weigh-in.

As it turned out, my weight was still within the range handled by the office scale, sparing me the additional embarrassment and humiliation of having to trundle down to the local meat locker for a weigh-in there. Other than my substantial excess poundage that clung to my waist like I'd glued a massive inner tube to my midriff like the kind people use to float down lazy river rides, I passed the battery of tests with just less than flying colors.

Upon completing the physical, we got down to the nitty-gritty and discussed exactly why I could not be faithful to any of those best-selling diet plans on the market. The fact of the matter was, I explained to the good doctor, I could not forsake the foods I loved to eat, and I would not—and probably *could not*—make a point of weighing and measuring what food I could eat to the extent those programs suggested I had to. The way I figured it, there were no big mysteries or bizarre secrets to my supreme fatness.

What happened over the next fifteen or twenty minutes in that examination room would change not only my attitude toward losing weight but would have a profound—and lasting—effect on my life.

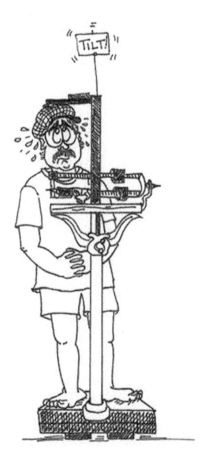

I stepped onto the gleaming white-black-and-silver Scales of Truth.

PART TWO

FIGHTING THE GOOD FIGHT

CHAPTER FIVE

DECLARATION OF WAR

The premise of the plan that was developed during that office visit, which would become the newfangled approach to losing weight, was really very basic. Those who love to eat and hate to exercise do not have the innate self-discipline to give up the food they enjoy. Nor do they have the inherent determination and drive to begin exercising, so there is very little hope that any of them can be completely true to the mandates of those diets. Well, guess what? You can have your cake and eat it too! That bears repeating: you can have your cake and eat it too. That was the revelation that forever altered my life.

The principles of this weight-loss plan to better eating and a happier lifestyle—which are discussed in detail in the next chapter—not only permit you to eat whatever you want but actually encourage you to. "No way!" you exclaim in utter disbelief. This approach doesn't just encourage you to do that; it *insists* upon it! The beautiful thing is, you'll lose weight in a steady, healthy manner that is conducive to keeping it off—in spite of yourself.

Chances are, you'll discover that, as you design and implement your personal agenda under the program, your energy level will increase to the point that you'll actually begin to exercise more—not because you have to but because you'll want to.

By following this plan, I lost more than thirty pounds in just over three months. By the end of the fourth or fifth week, my energy level increased to the point where I actually wanted to get out and be more active than I was accustomed to being. Of course, almost *any* activity was more than I was accustomed to. About six weeks into following the plan, my waistline had noticeably slimmed, and I hadn't given up a single item of food that I enjoyed eating. Not one. It was absolutely incredible.

Any war can be won if the battle plan is well conceived and implemented precisely. This program is a carefully planned blueprint for success in fighting the war on overeating. By following the attack plans described in the next chapter, you will be waging a war against your waistline that you can *actually win*—once and for all.

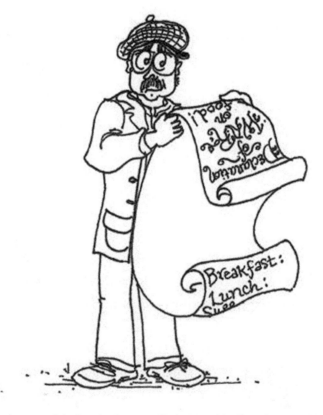

Any war can be won if the battle plan is well conceived and implemented precisely.

There are no gimmicks or insane schemes involved. If you approach the battle with the same fervor and resolve and in the same fashion I did, you'll simply be making common-sense decisions concerning your eating habits, and ultimately, you'll find yourself sneaking around. Only this time, you'll surprise yourself by sneaking around to exercise, rather than for extra food. The whole plan is simple and sensible—the way things really ought to be.

The diet books got to be so ridiculous with their demands that I didn't know whether to laugh or cry. Instead, I ate a whole bunch of comfort food. You know the kind I'm talking about: anything sweet and tasty.

I just had a real issue with measuring out and weighing so much of this meat and that vegetable or looking up and writing down the number of calories I had eaten for that particular meal. Besides, it wasn't always easy to find out how many calories were crammed into a couple of Big Macs and large fries back in the day. It just seemed incredibly petty, you know? Plus, it was really, really boring. I knew I wouldn't bother to do any of it after a few weeks or days or—heck, who am I kidding—hours. I'd be forever banished to another dimension, where fat folks who failed to fulfill the rules of dieting were left to roam aimlessly like zombies.

But there is hope for you. You can lose the weight you've always wanted to, and you can do it in a way that is healthy and sound and actually fosters keeping the weight off once you've reached your goal.

As I've already mentioned, this approach does not require you to do any "heavy lifting," like many of the diet plans you may be familiar with. There are no foods to give up, weigh, measure, or count. You won't have to exercise unless you want to. All you have to do is follow the attack plans and have the resolve to follow through with them. That's it.

So, with that said, it's time to put on your armor, grab your ammunition, and go to war!

CHAPTER SIX

BUILDING THE WAR CHEST

T o fight any war, you must build a war chest that gives you the strength to win. Altogether, there are six plans of attack that form the heart and soul—the war chest—of the campaign you'll undertake in this weight-loss war. For the most part, the concepts described are not necessarily original or revolutionary principles. However, a few have been tweaked a bit—especially where it was necessary to break down barriers that may get in your way—to help you persevere as you fight the good fight.

What you need most as you begin your journey is a nudge in the right direction. So for starters, these little tweaks are designed to help you develop the *will* and the will*power* to redefine the way you eat and the lifestyle you live. This notion is certainly not unique by any means, but it addresses one of the main drawbacks to dieting.

Then, to address another issue with conventional dieting, there is an attack plan that is actually unique and really is the cornerstone of the program. It's your own pot of gold at the end of the rainbow, which appears at the end of each week. Look at it as a just reward for all the fighting you've done during the previous seven days. You need that frequent and consistent gratification to reassure you that you're doing the right thing.

One thing traditional diet plans don't really make clear is this: how long is the dieting going to last? With this program, there is an attack plan that assists you in determining just how long you want—or need—to follow the regimen to reach your desired weight.

The last attack plan provides you with a healthy dose of courage to help you through the battle you're about to wage. This attack plan shares with you seven tips to keep you focused on the good fight. These tips are intended to ease you through a few of the obstacles that might occur.

Without further ado, here are the plans of attack that build the war chest that can change your life completely.

Attack Plan I:
Visit Your Physician and Get a Physical

This could be the only common link between this approach to losing weight and those run-of-the-mill diet plans, but it is absolutely imperative that you do it. Go see your family doctor or health-care professional, and get a physical. If, according to your doctor, the only malady you actually suffer from is a voracious and insatiable appetite, then tip the scales and move on to the next attack plan.

It is absolutely crucial to have a candid discussion with your physician, one in which a consensus is reached and you communicate your desires and needs. Make your physician a partner in your efforts, have him or her review your plan, and follow any advice that he or she may recommend.

In any event, remember that your health is at stake and should never be compromised under any circumstances.

Attack Plan II:
Weigh In and Set a Goal for Yourself

In order to achieve any type of success, you must have a vision and set reasonable goals as a means to measure your efforts periodically. In the case of a person trying to lose weight, the measurement part is pretty simple: all that has to be done is to get weighed. Now's as good a time as any. So pull out that bathroom scale, dust it off, and step up for the moment of truth.

Sure, you've already been weighed at the doctor's office as part of your physical examination, but aren't you curious to find out how big a difference there is between your scale and the one at the doctor's office? Besides, unless your doctor is insisting upon closely monitoring your progress, there's really no point in putting down big bucks to visit his or her office just to weigh in.

However, it is important to weigh yourself to gauge your progress. The key is to know *when* and *how often* to step on the scale. Recent reports suggest that weighing yourself daily is a good way to keep you on top of any weight fluctuations. This program recommends that you weigh yourself only once a month.

Why the difference? Well, the temptation to tip the scale all too frequently when trying to lose weight is a powerful one, and doing it more than once a month could adversely affect your resolve. Most people don't generally want to do this diet thing to begin with, so it's just natural to look for reasons to give up. Not seeing immediate results is one of the best reasons to beat the dream of a nice, lean body to within an inch of its life and kill what little resolve you may have.

If you ask a hundred dieters whether they've ever given up because they couldn't resist the temptation of the almighty scale, nearly every one of them would probably raise their hands. Well, listen carefully: immediate results are not going to happen. So do yourself a favor and hide your bathroom scale. If you weigh yourself too often, you'll only become despondent or angry or discouraged at the apparent lack of progress you're making. It's a fact.

As for *when* you should weigh yourself, the best time is generally at the start of your day, before you've eaten or dressed. This makes the most sense, because you may actually gain weight throughout the day because of variations in food and fluid consumption. The real key is to weigh yourself at the same time of day whenever you do weigh yourself. Consistency counts here.

So go on, step on the scale and let the numbers flash before your very eyes. Write the weight down on a piece of paper and put it in a safe place. I actually taped mine on the refrigerator door as a not-so-subtle reminder of my mission.

Now have someone hide the scale. If it's hidden away, that's one less thing lying around to stub your toe on. Just don't leave it somewhere convenient where it is liable to tempt you.

Now that you know where you stand weight-wise, and having consulted your friendly physician previously, you should have a firm idea of how much excess baggage you need to leave behind on the weight-loss carousel to be at *your* ideal weight. And what, precisely, is your ideal weight? Good question.

Remember those charts mentioned awhile back? For what it's worth, they do merit some consideration when determining what your ideal weight should be. Funny, though, it seems these weight-chart people can't agree on things either, judging from articles that have been published through the years. Get your hands on one of those charts and look at it. Then throw it away.

The truth is, your ideal weight will become self-apparent as you drop the pounds. When you reach a certain point, you'll know that you're at the weight you're supposed to be. Maybe you'll look in the mirror and smile at that attractive, slender figure reflecting back. Perhaps it'll be as simple as an old friend, amazed at your new slender self, smiling and saying, "Wow! You look really great!" Maybe it's just a feeling you have. But you'll know when you've reached your ideal weight, one way or another. This you can count on.

Of course, for the sake of establishing a goal for yourself, you need guidance and direction in the how-much-weight-do-I-really-need-to-lose-to-be-fit decision. If your doctor is as insightful and helpful as mine was, he'll probably put his two cents' worth into the matter by telling you about where you should be weight-wise. You can use that as your goal. After all, your doctor is the professional.

If you're still uncertain about whether you really have the gumption and wherewithal to see this approach through, do this: find a full-length mirror that affords you some privacy. Get stark naked and gaze at your reflection. Now close your eyes and imagine the leaner, more fit person you want to—and *can*—be! If you're still not visualizing that beautiful outer you, close your eyes and click your heels together three times. Then repeat, "There *is* a slender me. There *is* a slender me. There *is* a slender me." That helped Dorothy in *The Wizard of Oz* to get what she wanted, so who's to say it wouldn't work for you? Of course, she *did* have ruby slippers.

Seriously, though, try to imagine that sleeker, leaner you; then open your eyes. Which image makes you feel better? Ruby slippers or no, you have the power to change—you've had it all the time. You *can* be that slender person you saw in your mind's eye.

If you are like me, the realization that I had a ton—okay, it wasn't *quite* that much—of weight to lose was pretty darned shocking, not to mention depressing. Troubling though that revelation was, I knew I had to get my rather substantial fanny in gear and do something. So I set the wheels in motion with this plan.

The following chart illustrates the basic concept of this weight-loss program. The whole plan is focused on the amount of time it will take to lose the weight you'd like.

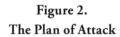

Figure 2.
The Plan of Attack

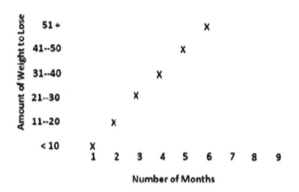

Note: If you have an excessive amount of weight to lose—fifty or more pounds—you should schedule a series of appointments with your physician or health-care professional to allow for professional guidance and monitoring over the extended length of following this program.

The plan is designed for about a ten-to-twelve-pound loss each month, give or take a pound or two. As a rule of thumb, you can figure it will take you about one month for every ten pounds you want to trim off your weight.

On your calendar, count off the number of months consistent with your intended weight loss. Find the corresponding date to today's date within that month. Put a great big star on that day. That's your V-W Day. This is the day you declare your victory over weight!

Attack Plan III:
Plan Your Personal Agenda and Strategy

If there really is a difficult part to this plan of mine, this must be it. You have to start someplace, and this is the beginning. This weapon requires you to analyze what—and how much—you eat over the course of a week, as well as *when* you eat, which is pretty important too. Before you respond with, "Oh, I knew there was a catch," remember, there's no heavy labor stuff to this.

You do have to be honest about laying out your personal agenda if you are seriously committed to losing weight on this program. Writing things down is a good way to be honest with ourselves, since our memories can often trick us. When you think about it, there is absolutely no reason not to be, since this list you'll put together can be secreted away so that nobody ever sees it. If you just refuse to trust anybody at all, you could carry the list with you.

Over the course of the program, you will log what you ate, when you ate it, and how much food you actually consumed. Each of these factors is critical in changing your eating habits and in developing the willpower it takes to eat healthier and more wisely.

In today's computerized world, it is far easier to compose and keep the list you prepare. A basic format is easy to set up as a table in a Microsoft Word document or an Excel spreadsheet. If you're computer savvy enough, you can create a folder to keep the information in and make the files password protected, if you so choose. A copy of the following form is included at the end of the book.

Figure 3.
Daily Analysis Sheet

WEEK		DATES		DAY	
MEAL	WHAT I ATE			AMT	TIME OF DAY

Key: B = Breakfast L = Lunch D = Dinner S = Snack

As shown in the above figure, you will be tracking the essentials of your eating patterns for each day.

To begin, you need to identify the week you're completing. Directly beside the **WEEK** box, enter the number corresponding to the number of the week you're logging. For example, your first week will be entered as **1**, and so on. In the space next to the **DATES** box, enter the calendar dates covered by the week; for example, **04/01–04/07**. Indicate the day of the week in the space next to the **DAY** box. For ease of reference, you may want to coordinate analysis week dates with the week dates on the calendar you used to indicate your V-W date.

Figure 4.
The Date Line

WEEK		DATES		DAY	

Under the **MEAL** heading, list which meal or snack you are referring to. This is indicated simply by a **B** for breakfast, **L** for lunch, **D** for dinner, and **S** for snack.

Figure 5.
The Meal Column

MEAL	WHAT I ATE	AMT	TIME OF DAY
B			
L			
D			
S			

In the **WHAT I ATE** column, make an itemized list of everything you ate for that particular meal or snack. Be as specific as you can to ensure that you remember the details. Repeat this listing for each meal and snack you have on any given day.

Figure 6.
The What I Ate Column

MEAL	WHAT I ATE	AMT	TIME OF DAY
B			
L			
D			
S			

Before going any further, there are a few preliminaries to discuss. References are made to servings and to serving sizes that need to be defined more clearly. For discussion's sake, a serving refers to the number of times you partake of the dishes being presented for consumption. For example, you may begin your evening meal by helping yourself to meat, potatoes, and a side vegetable, along with a dessert. That represents *one* serving, no matter how much of each you put on your plate.

The Hand That Feeds You

Serving size, on the other hand, is the *amount* of each food you put on your plate to constitute each serving. Let the hand that feeds you also be your guide in how much food that is going to be.

Figure 7 on the following page is provided to give you an idea of how much of something is just about right to be a "normal" serving. But allow me to offer you a "helping hand."

To determine a normal serving, begin by looking at the open palm (including fingers) of your hand. Whether you're having meat, fish, or poultry, your selection should be no larger than the size of your open palm. That's a normal-sized serving.

Now clench your fist. Any food that is doled out with a serving spoon should not contain a larger amount than the size of your closed fist. Whether it's cereal, potatoes, or rice, as well as certain canned or frozen vegetables, you should follow this guideline.

Why use this type of measurement over the scale and conventional meauring cups or spoons? For one thing, it's a heck of a lot easier unless you plan to carry around all that stuff wherever you go. The reality is also that no two bodies are exactly alike. So it follows that differing body masses and weights translate into different requirements for nutrition and nourishment. Explained simply, a person who has a "bigger frame" will usually need more sustenance than a person who is considerably smaller. So it makes sense to use these built-in tools to measure your *personal* normal serving sizes.

These are not exact measurements, but that's part of the point. Let the hand that feeds you also be your guide when determining *how much* you should eat.

Figure 7.
What Is a "Normal" Serving?

1 Serving Spoon	Fist-Sized
Meat/Fish	Palm-Sized, including Fingers
Sandwich	2 Slices of Bread/Toast
Potato/Snack Chips	Approximate Serving Listed on Bag
Cereal	Fist-Size
Eggs (Any Style)	2 Medium/Large Eggs
Bacon/Sausage	2 Slices/Links or 1 Patty
Pancakes	2 Medium Cakes/3 Small Cakes
Ice Cream	Fist-Sized

*Any food that has a recommended serving listed on its container should be approximated closely to that serving recommendation.

A normal serving would be one piece of meat, fish, or poultry that is about the size of the palm of your hand or one fist-sized helping of casserole or whatever serves as the "main dish," as well as a fist-sized amount each of potatoes and a side vegetable, if they are included as part of the meal. The same is true with the helping of dessert. If you're piling on the number of times you plop a spoonful on your plate, you're exceeding a normal serving.

If you really feel like splurging, eat fresh vegetables, such as broccoli, carrots, squash, green beans, or asparagus, to help fill you up. I've discovered that all of these vegetables are actually quite good when steamed or grilled. They also make a tasty—and healthy—vegetable medley when mixed together.

To guide you further on your journey to eating healthier and more wisely, refer to—and study—figure 1 in chapter 1 to get sound advice on what and how much to eat during the course of a week. The information is particularly valuable.

In the **AMT** column, you will enter the number of *normal servings* you helped yourself to during your various meals and snacks. During the early weeks of your analysis, you may find yourself still dishing up more than your personal normal serving, if only because you're not yet thinking less is more. Be sure to enter anything over your personal normal serving as an additional helping.

When you indicate the amount, it is important to be consistent with your *definition* of that amount. For example, if you list a *4* in the **AMT** column to indicate the number of slices of bread to make two sandwiches, use that measurement throughout your analyses. Be consistent to keep things simple and easy to remember.

Figure 8.
The AMT Column

MEAL	WHAT I ATE	AMT	TIME OF DAY
B			
L			
D			
S			

Finally, be sure to enter *when* you're eating in the final column, **TIME OF DAY**. This is also crucial to the weight-loss endeavor. Our bodies are geared to burn calories as we move about during our day. In most cases, the later in the day we consume those calories, the less fat is going to burn off.

If, for example, you eat dinner at 6:00 p.m. and then sit in front of the television, those calories are going to stick with you a lot longer than those you accumulated at breakfast or lunch, provided, of course, that you live a reasonably active lifestyle. If, while watching evening television, you snack on high-caloric food and a little while later go to bed, you've not done anything to burn off those added calories.

Figure 9.
The Time of Day Column

MEAL	WHAT I ATE	AMT	TIME OF DAY
B			
L			
D			
S			

You need to prepare a separate sheet for each day. It is critically important that you keep as accurate a record for each meal, each day, as you possibly can. The weekly analysis is the basis from which you will draw your weight-loss attack plan. It is critical that you be honest about what you eat, how much you eat, and when you eat. Figure 10 on the next page shows a sample completed analysis.

You may be really surprised at just how much food you consumed during your day and week of analysis. Once you know how much you eat and when you eat it, the strategy is quite simple: over the course of the next few weeks, you are going to cut down—not *out*—what you've been accustomed to eating.

Figure 10.
Sample Completed Daily Analysis Sheet

WEEK	1	DATES	04/01–04/07	DAY	MONDAY

MEAL	WHAT I ATE	AMT	TIME OF DAY
B	toasted peanut butter sandwich	4	7:00A
	16 oz. whole milk	2	
	scrambled eggs	3	
S	12 oz. soda	1	9:15A
	candy bar	1	
L	baloney sandwich (ketchup/mustard)	2	12:00P
	potato chips (medium baggie)	1	
	12 oz. whole milk	1	
S	12 oz. soda	1	2:15P
	candy bar	1	
D	roast beef slices	3	6:00P
	mashed potatoes with gravy	3	
	peas	3	
	apple pie with ice cream	2	
	16 oz. whole milk	2	
S	apple pie with ice cream	2	9:30P
	16 oz. soda	1	

Key: B = Breakfast L = Lunch D = Dinner S = Snack

Does the list cause a little voice inside of you to call out, "Oh, God! I'm going to be *sooo* hungry! I couldn't possibly cut down"?

The fact of the matter is, you *will* be hungry at first, but it's not as bad as it sounds. You can plan on feeling hungry for at least two to four days as you adjust your eating habits. But it won't be as bad as you may think, especially if you keep in mind *why* you're losing the weight: to feel better and live a healthier life.

An important thing to remember is that the hunger you're feeling isn't so much a biological *need* to eat as it is your mind making you *think* you're hungry because you're so accustomed to eating in a certain way. It's like psychological warfare, when you think about it. Be strong and fight the urges. It does get better rather quickly.

The whole key to success is to *reduce your consumption* based on your initial analysis but to do it *gradually.* This is how you train yourself to develop that rather elusive concept called willpower.

For example, if you discover that you have a real tendency to help yourself to three or four generous servings at dinnertime, during the first week of this program, you should strive to eliminate *just one* of those servings. Then, as your stomach is getting used to that idea, begin experimenting with cutting back on the *size* of the portion you dish out to yourself. In other words, by the end of week one, you'll be eating two or three servings—or whatever is one less than your analysis—instead of three or four. At the same time, rather than taking a mammoth glob of, for example, mashed potatoes along with everything else being served, you will reduce it to just a "normal" glob.

What must be done is simple: you have to coax yourself gradually, so you can get used to the idea of eating less, not just jump right into it. It's similar to the notion of sticking your toes in the water before diving right in. This approach teaches you how to build up willpower over the course of three, even four or five weeks. The hand-holding helps. It helped me. It can and will help you.

Attack Plan IV:
The Pot of Gold at the End of the Rainbow

I needed an incentive that meant something—something a bit more instantly gratifying than just the end-result weight loss—if I was to achieve my lofty goal of losing seventy-odd pounds. Thus, while most diets are long-range, long-term in their process, this particular method shrinks and compresses the whole concept into weeklong sections— coincidentally about as long as my diet-related attention span—and provides a real, honest-to-goodness incentive that you can sink your teeth into. Literally.

Stop and think for a moment. What is your absolute favorite treat? Mine's ice cream and lots of it. I swear I cannot live without it. I believed that unless I found some sort of avant-garde diet plan that incorporated lots of ice cream in its regimen, I was destined to slip and slide and fall from its good graces. Unless I got my ice cream fix through the marvels of some outrageous new diet scheme, I was going to lose the Battle of the Bulge before I could really begin. No doubt about it.

The great thing about this plan is that it is designed to allow for that mental struggle with your favorite treat. You can eat it. Unheard of? Absolutely! Revolutionary? Not at all. It's just common sense.

Ask yourself this question: would you work at a job that you hated— or loved, for that matter—without accepting an occasional paycheck? Probably not. More often than not, that's what really motivates a person to go to work, to get that paycheck at the end of the designated pay period.

Quite frankly, there is absolutely no reason under the sun to forgo your favorite treat just because you're trying to lose weight. Rather, your treat is your "gastronomical paycheck" for a job well done. It is your pot of gold at the end of the rainbow, if you will.

If you faithfully follow the strategy you set up in Attack Plan III, you should be rewarded for your honest effort at the end of the week, just like when you're working. After all, that *is* what dieting is, a tremendous amount of work. At least it seemed that way to me.

The subtle changes in eating habits, which are implemented early in the plan, are designed to foster success. Of course, every day you follow your personal agenda is a shot of encouragement, followed by a long draw on the elixir of self-respect.

I found that during the initial week, I had no difficulty being faithful to the personal agenda I had planned. I was enthusiastic about the prospect of succeeding at it and completely convinced that I could do the weight-loss thing without starving myself. Besides, I knew there was the matter of a reward for my efforts just a scant few days away. As I got further into my strategy, my appetite and the thoughts of a little more food were suppressed sufficiently enough that just a quick flash of that reward—in my case, it was a half-pint of my favorite ice cream—diverted my attention long enough for the urge to cheat to slither away. Of course, no one is perfect.

I discovered that the one time I did cheat during the week, I couldn't bring myself to order the ice cream. I walked right up to the girl at the counter, slapped the money down, but I just couldn't get the words out of my mouth. I simply did an about-face and marched straight out the door. I even forgot to pick up the money I'd laid on the counter. Honest.

I'm basically an honest person, and even if I weren't, the last person I would ever want to cheat would be myself. I truly believe that people who are willpower-challenged looking into this plan feel the same way. To thine own self be true. It's human nature.

Attack Plan IV is simply about setting a reward for yourself. It is an essential ingredient to succeeding in the Battle of the Bulge. After a week of being completely faithful to the strategy of the approach, treat yourself to something really, really tasty. You earned it. Just remember not to go overboard with the amount. Keep it sensible. As hard as it may be to believe, this method of rewarding yourself *weekly* really does work. I couldn't have succeeded without it.

Attack Plan V:
Effecting the Strategy

There are certain foods you know you should avoid. It seems every time you watch a news program or read the newspaper, some new study has come out with still *another* kind of food you should forget about eating. The list seems practically endless. It seems the only foods those research people want you to eat are those veggie-type things. Yuck!

Still, there has been a lot of time and money spent on researching this, so they *must* know what they're talking about. But don't you find it more than just slightly curious that the foods they claim offer no nutritional value whatsoever are only those types of food that are really sweet and taste really good?

The point remains, there are certain foods you know you should avoid. The problem generally is that you just don't *want* to. You know what you like, and you'll usually eat it.

Most diet plans preach that you absolutely, positively must cut out this type of food or that kind of food to lose weight. There are programs that insist you eat a low-protein, no-fat diet to lose weight and be healthy. Others extol the virtues of a low- or no-carb diet as being the better and healthier way to diet.

When I first set out on my quest to find the "perfect" diet, I read as many books as I could find on the subject. At that time, there weren't many. One, *The Doctor's Quick Weight Loss Diet* by Dr. Irwin Maxwell Stillman—commonly known as the Stillman Diet, which was published in 1967—promoted a diet rich in meat, fish, eggs, cheeses, and spices. However, it did not allow the follower to eat fats or carbohydrates, including vegetables and fruits. While quick weight loss did occur, further research showed a lack of nutritional balance. This led to certain vitamin deficiencies that could cause adverse health effects.

In 1972, Dr. Robert Atkins published his *Diet Revolution*, which extolled a low-carb diet. This program permitted the follower to eat fatty foods that were thought to be off-limits to dieters but could result in a fifteen-pound weight loss over a two-week period. According to the Atkins Diet, the body is like an engine and needs constant fuel. The body typically draws from stored carbohydrates to supply that fuel. By all but removing carbs, the body is forced to use stored fats as its source of fuel, which results in shedding pounds.

One of the issues with the diet, however, was that, while it did have tremendous short-term success, it was difficult to maintain in the long-term. As with the Stillman Diet, Atkins's plan also came up lacking in the area of balanced nutrition.

The bottom line is the Stillman and Atkins plans, as well as others, fell short of offering a "perfect" diet.

As research into nutrition and health has matured through the years, several other weight-loss plans have emerged. Two of the most notable programs, Weight Watchers® and NutriSystem®, provide plans that encourage better eating habits through their prepared foods and support networks. While weight-loss results can be extremely dramatic, the fact that the follower must pay—whether for a membership or for monthly prepared foods, or both—can be cost-prohibitive. Although potentially very effective, not everyone has the financial resources to participate in these types of weight-loss programs. But you can achieve success without spending any more money than you would under your current situation.

The answer to effective weight loss is really very simple. All you need to do is *moderate* your consumption.

In that office visit with Dr. Hepner so many years ago, he provided me with a list of foods that I needed to moderate if I were to seriously attempt to lose weight:

✓potatoes	✓corn	✓butter
✓cheese	✓bread	✓candy
✓whole milk	✓pastries	✓ice cream

For those health-conscious believers in the purveyors of unpleasant news as it relates to eating, I *could* say that this list went on and on. But I won't, because, quite honestly, that was it. The truth is, though, with the last two items—the pastries and the ice cream—he may as well have told me he'd have to sew my mouth shut for me to lose weight.

Be that as it may, the kind doctor just rattled off those few items and explained that everyone should monitor their consumption of starchy foods in particular. He added that if I made an honest effort to control my binges on these particular items, I would have no trouble losing weight. As it turned out, he was right.

The important thing to remember is that the operative word here is *moderate*—not give up or cut out. I could certainly handle that.

For the record, I love every single item on that list, and if he had told me to give up even one of them, it probably would have been another good reason to find a different doctor or just resign myself to being overweight. No way would I be willing to sacrifice any of the foods that made up the bulk of my diet. Besides, everybody knows you can't teach an old dog new tricks. Right?

So how do you go about moderating your consumption? If you've followed the attack plans up to now, you've pretty much already outlined how you're going to do it. But to outline a program carefully and to really implement the change are two vastly different matters, right? Wrong. There is no secret to it. There is no mystery. All you have to do from here on is *gradually* reduce the number of portions you help yourself to, while *gradually* reducing the size of servings you take. Sound familiar?

The Implementation Process

The premise of the implementation process is very basic. It is set up similar to the technique that was described in Attack Plan II. This is intentional. The more weight you have to lose, the more time you need to bring your eating habits under control.

As figure 11 below illustrates, if you are trying to lose roughly thirty pounds, your agenda should reflect the full extent of your change— that's the reduction in consumption—by the end of the third or fourth week. If you are attempting to lose forty pounds or so, your agenda needs to stretch to a fourth or fifth week; with fifty-plus pounds, your reduction in consumption should extend to six or seven weeks, and so on. The thing is, you need to take your time making these reductions, to ensure your success in losing weight.

Figure 11.
The Implementation Process

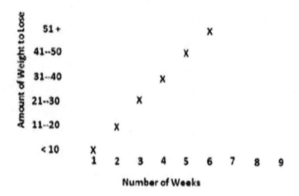

The number of weeks necessary to reduce your consumption of food should correspond to the amount of weight you want to lose. For example, if you wish to lose forty pounds, reduce the amount of food you eat over a four- or five-week period.

Again, in cases of extreme amounts of weight to be lost, the agenda you create should be reviewed by your physician or health-care professional and monitored on a regular basis. To do otherwise could be harmful to your overall health. Work your plan so that it takes you down the weight-loss path without causing you to stumble and fall.

The point is that you should modify your eating habits gradually, with the least amount of resistance from your stomach and your mind. It will be far more difficult to do that in the early days and weeks of the agenda, as you retrain your mind and begin shrinking your stomach, so bite off only what you can comfortably chew early on.

However you go about changing your eating habits, don't get carried away with doing too much too soon, because it simply will not work. You may lose lots and lots of weight quickly, but you could also seriously affect your health doing things that way. Conversely, you could end up doing great that way—which is to say, *starving* yourself—for three or four days or a week and then, all of a sudden you'll get hit with a tremendous urge to binge, and you'll start eating. And eating. And eating. So banish the thought of instant weight loss. It just won't work.

I knew going in at the start of each week exactly how much I had eaten the previous week, and I kept envisioning where I wanted to be consumption-wise by the end of that week.

Breakfast

I'd generally begin my day with a hearty breakfast. After all, the experts always advised that it was the most important meal of the day. So, of course, wanting to follow good, solid advice, I ate a big breakfast each day. Typically, I would eat three or four peanut butter sandwiches on toast—that's six to eight *slices* of bread—or two bowls of cereal and one or two sandwiches, washed down with two or three tumblers of ice-cold milk. There were days when I opted for three or four fried eggs and three or four slices of toast smothered in butter. That occurred when I was thinking more health-consciously, though.

Lunch

My eating habits at lunchtime were pretty routine. I'd prepare two sandwiches of virtually any processed meat—smothered in mayonnaise or some other garnish—slice up a lot of cheese, and add a generous portion of potato chips on the side. I'd generally consume at least one twelve-ounce soda, but when I was especially thirsty, I'd treat myself to a second one. On those days when I really felt like treating myself, I'd take myself to lunch at the local diner and feast on whatever met my fancy: a bowl of chili; a couple of cheeseburgers; maybe even one substantial serving of my personal favorite, macaroni and cheese. Mind you, this was *in addition to* eating my packed lunch more times than not.

Dinner

After a hard day of physical labor, my appetite at dinner was always voracious. I would eat at least three, if not four, tremendous helpings of everything served. Mountains of potatoes, awash in a sea of gravy; enormous portions of meat; and lots and lots of peas or corn, those being the only vegetables I liked. It usually required two or three large glasses of whole milk to satisfy my thirst at dinner. And, oh yes, if a dessert was prepared, as it routinely was, I would insist on eating two generous helpings of it.

Snacks

Here's the really great part. My snacking was virtually nonstop during the day and night. But in my defense, the experts say that one should "graze" throughout the day. So that's what I did. In the morning, I'd munch on a sweet roll and drink plenty of milk. For added energy in the afternoon, I could almost always be seen with a candy bar in one hand and a soda in the other. In the evening, while watching television, I'd eat a bowl of ice cream—usually four or five heaping scoops—or a dozen cookies or so dunked in a glass of milk. If dessert had, in fact, been served at dinner, you can bet I cleaned it out that night, more times than not. Sometimes, if I was really hungry, a sandwich or two would precede the snack and, no matter what, I always drank at least one sixteen-ounce soda every evening.

Please remember that this is a glimpse at my first week of analysis. The actual list was kept very accurately, recording the time of day that I ate and how much food I shoved in my mouth at one sitting.

I have included a random selection of the daily logs I accumulated during my weight-loss odyssey to illustrate the recommended way to complete each day's consumption. There is one for the preliminary week's analysis and one day for each of the first three weeks of my personal agenda.

Figure 12.
Typical Preliminary Daily Analysis

WEEK	PA	DATES	03/25–03/31	DAY	MONDAY

MEAL	WHAT I ATE	AMT	TIME OF DAY
B	toasted peanut butter sandwich	4	7:00A
	16 oz. whole milk	2	
	scrambled eggs	3	
S	12 oz. soda	1	9:15A
	sweet roll	2	
L	baloney sandwich (ketchup/mustard)	2	12:00P
	potato chips (medium baggie)	1	
	cheddar cheese slices	8	
	12 oz. whole milk	1	
S	12 oz. soda	1	2:15P
	candy bar	1	
D	roast beef slices	3	6:00P
	mashed potatoes with gravy	3	
	peas	3	
	apple pie with ice cream	2	
	16 oz. whole milk	2	
S	apple pie with ice cream	2	9:30P
	16 oz. soda	1	

Key: B = Breakfast L = Lunch D = Dinner S = Snack

Looking back, I confess that I am truly shocked and appalled at the amount of food I was consuming in a day's time. Yes, I am gravely ashamed of myself. But those are the indisputable facts, and it certainly is a graphic illustration of why I was overweight back then.

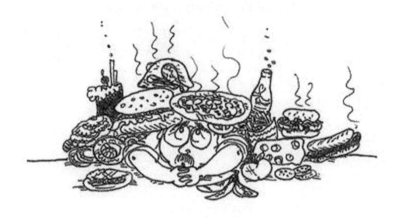

I confess that I am truly shocked and appalled at the
amount of food I was consuming in a day's time.

After weighing in and discussing my weight objectives with my doctor,
my goal was to lose just over seventy pounds, so I planned my personal
agenda to last just over eight weeks.

Week One

I'll begin by confessing to something up front: during those first three
or four days, there were tremendous hunger pangs pounding away at
the insides of my stomach. But each time I was ready to concede and
give in to those dastardly urges, I closed my eyes and pictured how great
that ice cream—every sumptuous, delicious bite of the half-pint—was
going to taste at the end of the week. It managed to console me and
placate my rampant urges. Sweet inspiration.

The point here is that no matter how dreadfully those urges are
banging away in your stomach, they will eventually go quietly in the
good night. Well, maybe not so quietly, but they will dissipate after a
few days. I promise. So don't let them beat you at this. Think pleasant
gastronomical thoughts to chase the pangs away.

As I prepared my personal agenda, I kept in mind that my consumption-reduction plan had to be gradual in order to succeed. I evaluated what and when I ate during my analysis week. I also reviewed how much I ate. Then I put together a personal agenda that I believed I could stick to and ultimately begin reducing my consumption. The following is a summary of the agenda I created.

Breakfast

The three or four peanut butter sandwiches dwindled to two by the third morning of week one. When I opted for the healthier repast of eggs, my limit was three—scrambled—with no more than two pieces of toast to complement them. I still drank milk, but no more than one glass, compensating with coffee or water instead. During the first week, when I ate cereal, it was still two bowls but without the sandwich chaser.

Lunch

The week started with the unceremonious dispatch of the chips and cheese from my lunchtime meal. The third day of week one marked the trimming of the second sandwich to a mere half, so that by the end of the week, I was eating one whole sandwich as my luncheon mainstay. I also restricted myself to only one soda, no matter what. On those occasions when I felt like treating myself by drifting into the diner for a hot meal, I eliminated my prepacked lunch by casting it into the trash on my way out of the factory door. It was a tough thing to do, but I did it—with only a hint of remorse.

Dinner

Common sense led me to believe that this meal would be the most difficult to alter, so I had to really plan my attack carefully. I began the week by reducing the *size* of my portions. Then, on the fourth day, I made the plunge by killing the urge to help myself to more than three servings. On the sixth and seventh days, I limited myself to two helpings of dinner—just to prepare myself *mentally* for what lay ahead. I drank milk but would substitute water for a second glass. As for any dessert served, I permitted myself a very substantial portion, but only *one*.

Snacks

Where—and *what*—to cut out? I essentially attempted to trick myself mentally for the first few days. I substituted several cookies for that one morning sweet roll. It was the familiar "the-more-the-merrier" routine, only set to food. I started out by giving myself eight small cookies and reduced the number by one every day. Perhaps the most difficult task I faced that first week was my decision to eliminate that afternoon candy bar—my energy booster. I settled for the rush of an ice-cold soda, drinking lots of water to stave off the midday demon hunger pangs. Another little trick I used was to chew a lot of gum to keep my mouth busy as I attempted to trim the candy from my snacking routine. It really worked. As for the evening snack, I made the decision right away to relegate the nightly soda to an every-other-night treat—it served as a mini-reward for doing well. What I discovered, rather interestingly, over the course of the week was that the nighttime snack was less of an issue than I had anticipated. Beginning with a bunch of cookies, coupled with the leftover dessert, by the end of the week, I'd managed to cut back to one or the other, but never both. Again, water became a very good substitute for my desire to constantly snack on food.

Oh yes, I did eat a half-pint of my favorite ice cream at the end of the week. And I smiled after every single bite!

Figure 13.
Typical Week 1 Daily Analysis

WEEK	1	DATES	04/01–04/07	DAY	MONDAY
MEAL	WHAT I ATE			AMT	TIME OF DAY
B	scrambled eggs			3	7:00A
	toast			2	
	16 oz. whole milk			1	
	coffee			2	
S	cookies			8	9:15A
	coffee or water			2	
L	baloney sandwich (ketchup/mustard)			1½	12:00P
	12 oz. whole milk			1	
S	12 oz. soda			1	2:15P
D	baked chicken breasts			2	6:00P
	mashed potatoes with gravy			2	
	corn			1	
	cherry cobbler			1	
	16 oz. whole milk			2	
S	cherry cobbler			1	7:00P
	cookies			6	
	16 oz. soda			1	

Key: B = Breakfast L = Lunch D = Dinner S = Snack

Week Two

I began the week by reviewing what I had eaten, when I had eaten it, and the amount I had eaten during week one. I evaluated this information and formulated my eating plan for week two. As I did with the inaugural week, I created a very conservative reduction schedule to foster and encourage success, rather than developing a more aggressive plan that could have potentially resulted in failure. What I discovered was that something extraordinary occurred early in week two: my appetite had declined dramatically.

Breakfast

The two peanut butter sandwiches gave way to no more than one and a half sandwiches by the second day. My goal of eating only one sandwich by the end of the week was accomplished by day three. On those occasions when I elected to eat cereal instead of toast—my idea of balancing my diet, by the way—I was amazed to discover that one bowl more than filled me up.

Lunch

On the fourth day of the week, I leaped into action by substituting a generous portion of cottage cheese and a hard-boiled egg for my beloved sandwich and elected to drink a small amount of milk instead of the soda. For a couple of days, I felt I needed to eat half a sandwich, but by the end of the week, the mainstay of my midday feast was the cottage cheese—sometimes with sliced peaches to break up the blandness—and a hard-boiled egg. I resisted the temptation to take myself to lunch at the local restaurant, instead playing the mind-game routine of *envisioning* a hearty feast while scarfing down my cottage cheese. It wasn't perfect, mind you, but it got me through.

Dinner

Over the course of the week, I concentrated on further reducing the size of the portions I served myself. By midweek, I was controlling my appetite with two *average* servings of dinner, although I would often bypass seconds on everything but the main dish. Of course, I still had a very healthy helping of any dessert that was served.

Snacks

The urge for substantial evening snacks was dramatically diminished by the third or fourth day of week two. Whenever it was overwhelming, I would generally munch on three or four cookies with a small glass of milk to chase them down. Sometimes I would have an average-sized portion of the evening's dessert to mix up the epicurean routine. What I discovered was that on those nights when I drank my sixteen-ounce soda, no other snack was really necessary to quash the urges. Daytime snacks were virtually in the Smithsonian—like other significant matters of history. I had little need for a morning snack; in the afternoon, I was perfectly content with a twelve-ounce soda. That was it.

Because I'd been such a good boy and followed my personal agenda faithfully, at the end of the week I ate a half-pint of my favorite ice cream, smiling after each delightful spoonful and harboring no guilt whatsoever.

Figure 14.
Typical Week 2 Daily Analysis

WEEK	2	DATES	04/08–04/14	DAY	WEDNESDAY	
MEAL	WHAT I ATE			AMT	TIME OF DAY	
B	Wheaties with whole milk			1	7:00A	
	16 oz. whole milk			1		
L	cottage cheese			1	12:00P	
	hard-boiled egg			1		
	baloney sandwich (ketchup/mustard)			½		
	12 oz. whole milk			1		
S	12 oz. soda			1	2:15P	
D	baked chicken breasts			2	6:00P	
	mashed potatoes with gravy			2		
	corn			1		
	cherry cobbler			1		
	16 oz. whole milk			2		
S	cookies			4	7:30P	
	12 oz. whole milk			1		

Key: B = Breakfast L = Lunch D = Dinner S = Snack

Week Three

Week three represented the summit of the mountain for me, just as you will reach the week when your personal agenda really begins working for you. Once you reach the summit, it's all downhill from there. No longer will the urges haunt you and tug at your tummy. You will have significantly diminished your level of consumption, ideally to an *average* one. You will find your appetite—and your stomach—shrinking. The really great thing is that you've been able to enjoy all those great foods you've always loved, including your weekly reward. Without it being dangled in front of me—especially in the early going—I would not have made it to this point.

After suffering through those two grueling weeks of modifying my consumption, I began week three with an amazing sense of confidence and a conviction that I was going to succeed. I felt better physically. I actually *wanted* to eat less and consequently drop the remaining weight. It was pretty much like nothing was going to stop me. That's all there was to it.

Breakfast

From three or four sandwiches at the outset, I had now altered my habit to the point that I was sometimes eating as little as one slice of toast, generously smeared with butter, and a couple of tumblers of milk. There were a couple of days during week three when I actually skipped breakfast altogether. What I discovered was that I would only eat when I was *hungry* and not simply because the food was there in front of me. This was absolutely the most significant change in my eating habits, as it turned out.

Lunch

By the end of the week, my lunch was consistently cottage cheese with an occasional hard-boiled egg. Once during the week, I treated myself to a soda instead of relying on milk as my beverage of choice. I also went out to the diner one day for lunch because—get this—I craved a salad. I kid you not. I still have a difficult time with that one, but it's true.

Dinner

Starting out the week, I was pretty much helping myself to two servings of everything, although I had a hard time finishing that second round. By the end of week three, I had successfully reduced my portions to one average serving. With that eaten, I'd often find myself contentedly patting or rubbing my stomach. As far as dessert went, you should know by now that I'm the type of guy who just cannot say no. Every time dessert was offered, I gladly accepted it. No question. No guilt.

Snacks

Other than my soda every other evening and an occasional craving for sweets, the urge to snack was pretty much out of the picture. If a quick flash in my mind of that half-pint of ice cream didn't subdue the craving, I'd eat two or three cookies. That was it. Another interesting personal phenomenon occurred during week three as well. I actually began munching on fruit as a substitute for the really sweet, sugary stuff. Near the end of the week, I got a really strong hankering to eat a banana, so I did—without feeling really weird about it. It actually tasted pretty good. For a *fruit*, I mean. Ultimately, bananas, peaches, pears, and strawberries became part and parcel of my personal agenda. There's not really much to say about my propensity for daytime snacking, except that it was virtually nonexistent. Other than an occasional soda or a banana, I just never felt the urge or had the *need*.

Figure 15.
Typical Week 3 Daily Analysis

WEEK	3	DATES	04/15–04/21	DAY	FRIDAY	
MEAL	WHAT I ATE			AMT	TIME OF DAY	
B	toast			1	7:00A	
	16 oz. whole milk			2		
L	cottage cheese with peach slices			1	12:00P	
	hard-boiled egg			1		
	12 oz. whole milk			1		
S	water			1	2:15P	
D	macaroni and cheese			1	5:30P	
	hot dog on a bun (ketchup/mustard)			1		
	16 oz. whole milk			2		
S	strawberries			1	8:00P	

Key: B = Breakfast L = Lunch D = Dinner S = Snack

Yes, of course, since I'd been a true-blue follower of my agenda and the approach for the whole week, I peacefully devoured that half-pint of ice cream—my just dessert for my efforts.

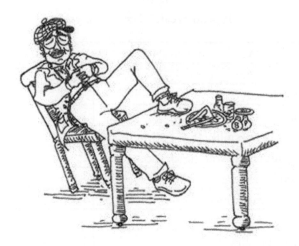

I'd often find myself contentedly patting or rubbing my stomach.

Summary

My personal agenda program continued for just over another four weeks. Once I'd reached the point of adjusting my eating habits to reflect my personal normal serving sizes, I was no longer fighting that psychological warfare that my mind formerly used to prey on me. When I had control over the cravings, I began eating healthier and more wisely. I became more physically active, and the weight loss became nearly effortless. I knew that I could finally realize that goal of losing just over seventy pounds.

Attack Plan VI:
Tips to Get You through the Struggles

When, in my frustration, I went and spoke with Dr. Hepner about losing weight, he essentially told me to use my judgment about things. He wanted me to quit working so darned hard at dieting and just do what felt right.

During the initial stages of trying to figure out what made sense to me, I fell into some typical traps, had to take a few steps back to evaluate the situation, and then made a few adjustments. This is the culmination of those efforts—what worked best to help me beat down the foe and lose the weight I never could before.

Since I suspect you will go through many of the same things I did, Attack Plan VI provides a few modest suggestions and reminders to help you get by those demon temptations which, by the way, you shouldn't confuse with that terrific Motown group from the '60s and '70s. They were great. These demon ones, not so much.

These seven tips are not original by any means. In fact, most of them have been recited—in one form or another—in many other books about weight loss. In actuality, they're really nothing more than a subtle dose of psychology, combined with simple common sense.

One thing to know about these suggestions is that they really can be quite effective. You should find them very useful in helping you through any weak moments or rough spots in your weight-loss journey.

Here they are, in no particular order of importance.

Tip 1:
LET YOUR INTUITION BE YOUR GUIDE
This is probably the *cardinal rule* of this approach. Let your intuition be your guide. If your intuition is telling you one thing, and your stomach is saying something different, then follow your intuition. Early in your assault against the demon of delicious desire, you are going to have to listen to a lot of rumblings and grumblings from your stomach. It'll be complaining—in its inimitable way— about the lack of sweet things you once passed off as nutritional substance. Ignore it. It's playing tricks with you. Instead, do what you intuitively believe is appropriate. Pay attention to your common sense. It will never steer you wrong. That's the guiding force in this program.

Tip 2:

EAT SLOWLY AND SAVOR EVERY BITE

Take your time eating, especially in the early stages of your personal agenda. Eating slowly has a way of tricking your mind *and* your stomach into believing you're eating more. I found that putting down my fork or spoon after each bite actually helped me chew my food more thoroughly, which actually aids in digestion. I only picked up one or the other after I'd swallowed the food in my mouth. I *felt* more satisfied. I don't profess to know why; I just know it works.

Tip 3:

VISUALIZE THE POT OF GOLD AT THE END OF THE RAINBOW

What are you to do when that constant thumping and yearning in your stomach escalates to the point of driving you to the fringe of madness—or worse yet, *cheating?* Relax. Close your eyes. Visualize. That very special pot of gold at the end of the rainbow is not *that* far from your reach, really. I cannot begin to explain how critical it was for me to know that I could reward myself at the end of a long, trying week of fighting off the demons. It really did keep me on track.

Tip 4:

GIVE YOURSELF A MINI-REWARD EVERY OTHER NIGHT TO KEEP YOU ON TRACK

If you just do not believe you are capable of lasting a whole week— after all, that's *seven* twenty-four-hour days— there's absolutely nothing wrong with rewarding yourself in a mini-fashion. If you feel the need, do what I did. After I cut out one of my routine evening snacks, I gave it back to myself every other day. If it's food rather than drink, reduce the normal serving by half. You'll feel better about things and still stay on the schedule you set on your personal agenda.

Tip 5:

TRY SUBSTITUTING GREAT-TASTING FRUIT LIKE BANANAS, APPLES, PEACHES, AND PEARS FOR COOKIES AND CAKES AND PIES

As I reduced my consumption of snack foods, I would occasionally experiment with fruit to see if my body could learn to accept unconditionally—and without fear of rejection— natural sweeteners, rather than stuff that amounted to nothing more than real sugar disguised as fake sugar. Not only did my body accept this fruit thing, but the fact of the matter is, I was completely surprised at how great it tasted. What I discovered was that one banana arrested the hunger pangs and tasted nearly as good as those cookies I was accustomed to eating, but with a lot fewer calories to worry about. Plus, I learned that experts declared them "good for you." That was all the endorsement I needed, I told myself. Things like sliced peaches or pears and canned fruit cocktail were personal favorites and helped change my snacking habits. Okay, it wasn't *fresh* fruit, but it *was* a start. A word of caution, though: not all canned fruit is preserved in its own natural juices. Many are actually doused in heavy corn syrup. Try to steer clear of the latter. But do try substituting fruit for the cookies and other baked goods you've been inclined to munch on. You may find that you actually like them, and it'll pay off in the long run.

Tip 6.

DON'T FIGHT THE FEELING TO GET OUT AND EXERCISE MORE WHEN YOUR ENERGY LEVEL INCREASES—AND IT WILL

I was amazed at how quickly my energy level increased once I began following this newfangled program. The amount of energy increase seemed directly proportional to the amount of consumption decrease. The less I ate, the more energetic and ambitious I became. So I got out and walked when I could have driven. I took stairs instead of riding the elevator or escalator. Things like that. Just don't fight the feeling. The exercise will help keep you focused on your mission. Plus, these strange things called endorphins will make you practically giddy over doing this whole exercise thing. I promise.

Tip 7:
KEEP YOURSELF BUSY
In other words, avoid the pitfalls of being idle. After all, "idle minds are the devil's workshop"—or so they say, right? Don't get caught up in feeding your idle time or boredom with food. Feed it, instead, with games, either mental or physical, or some sort of recreational activity. Just don't eat for the sake of eating. Call a friend and get away from the temptation. Do whatever it takes. This is extremely important advice, especially in the early going. You are going to experience tremendous urges that, without an occasional diversion, could beat you down and break you, causing you to give in. Don't do it. Find someone—or something—to keep you busy.

There you go, a few tips and reminders that will help keep you focused in your efforts to effect the various attack plans discussed and get you on your way to losing the weight you never thought you could.

Everybody's different, but if you put your heart into finding your pot of gold at the end of the rainbow every week, if you focus on your mission, and if you follow the lead of your common sense, you'll be able to eat what you want, strip off the pounds, and become more involved in recreational activities—and *life*. Believe me, exercising for fun is a heck of a lot better—and easier—than doing it because you have to. The keys to success are simple: reward yourself for your efforts each week, and rely on your intuition and common sense to lead you on your journey—and your effort to lose weight.

PART THREE

HOW THE WAR WAS WON

CHAPTER SEVEN

THE BATTLE OF THE BULGE

After toying with several diet plans for a number of weeks, and after a few false starts with the development of my own alternative plan, my personal Battle of the Bulge was launched in earnest in early 1971. With this fresh concept in mind, I set out to wage the war, somewhat dispirited by my past troubled campaigns against a formidable foe—my expanding waistline.

Relying on the attack plans I had developed and, armed with nothing more than a renewed determination, I marched blindly into the fray. My goal: drop just over seventy pounds and shed seven or eight inches from my waist.

I now know the meaning of the phrase "War is hell! The first four days were just that. That may sound overly dramatic, but as I trimmed my consumption level from three or four servings down to a mere two, hunger pangs battered at the pit of my stomach with an unrelenting pugilistic force like I'd never felt before. I prowled around the house, dodging the incoming attacks of snack food being hurled in my direction from the bunkers of the kitchen cabinets and the refrigerator.

Those initial nights were restless ones, spent tossing and turning as dreams led me through enchanted forests of hot-fudge sundaes and ice cream sodas; of chocolate layer cakes and hot apple pies. Mountains of mashed potatoes topped with melting butter were beckoning from beyond wide rivers of giblet gravy drifting lazily at the forest's edge.

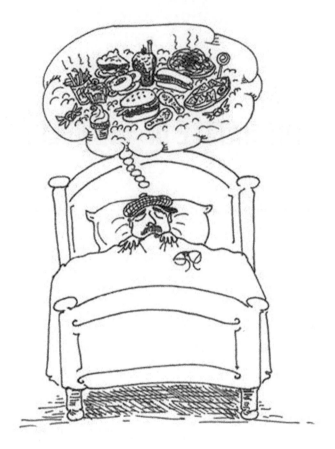

Those initial nights were restless ones, spent tossing and turning.

Under siege and feeling a bit downtrodden, I peered through cream-puff clouds and spotted a ray of hope: a rainbow, at the end of which was a magnificent pot of gold.

I suffered my first casualty of war on the fifth day of battle. A battalion of sweets, commanded by a tremendous cupcake, resorted to guerrilla war tactics and ambushed my camp, mining its perimeter. A piece of chocolate layer cake—passing itself off as a seemingly harmless *petit four*—besieged me and took me prisoner. Torture, torment, and humiliation ensued.

Left to my own devices and relying on common sense and a bit of the old true grit, I escaped from my captors, disguised as an immense Hostess Snowball. With only minor injuries to my pride, despite the deplorable conditions and my waning morale, I regrouped with a vow to return to battle with renewed vigor. I was not merely a survivor; I was fighting the good fight.

For three weeks, the war raged on, small victories claimed and celebrated with the ceremonial raising of the Baskin-Robbins banner each week as I savored the view from the summit.

Near the middle of that third week, I began feeling confident that the enemy lines were weakening. The counterattacks were less frequent, their force less dynamic. Victory was mine for the claiming and as sweet as a cinnamon roll fresh from the baker's oven.

After the first month of following this unconventional approach to losing weight, I stepped on the scales for the first time. Much to my surprise, I had lost eight pounds—even though I had spent the better part of three weeks rearranging my eating habits. I had hardly begun the war but was already eight pounds lighter. What had I sacrificed? I'd eaten everything that had been prepared and placed before me. I had rewarded myself with a half-gallon of my favorite ice cream during the month. Yet, here I was losing weight.

It was during the second month that my friends began commenting on my slimming waistline. The approach was essentially second nature. There were no more longing looks at the leftovers on the table; rather, I'd find myself contentedly patting my stomach after eating a meager portion—by my customary standards—of the grand repast.

Shortly before my second weigh-in, it occurred to me that I was actually eating more fruit than baked goods. It was absolutely astounding! How was such a thing possible?

What's more, I slipped on a pair of slacks that had once been ever so snug-fitting, only to discover that they still didn't fit well at all. Except this time, they were too big! When I took those slacks to be altered, they had to be taken in at the waist *over three inches.* "Holy moly!" I exclaimed to no one in particular. Man, I was so excited! I felt like I had finally *arrived.* My lifestyle and physical appearance were actually beginning to change, practically unbeknownst to me. It was pretty amazing stuff.

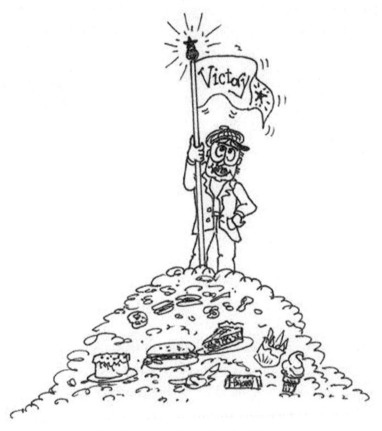

Small victories claimed and celebrated.

At the end of the second month on this absurd plan, I was surprised to discover that I had lost another thirteen pounds. That made twenty-one pounds in two months. Friends were telling me how great I looked.

Clothes had to be taken *in* to fit me! And another half-gallon of my favorite ice cream was devoured without guilt. Man, I was on a roll! I could hardly mask my excitement about life. It was nothing short of remarkable.

With the changes going on in my lifestyle, I discovered differences in my attitude and general approach to life. No longer looking or feeling frumpy, I experienced a resurgence of enthusiasm and energy. I was not only recharged, but supercharged! I bought new clothes. I walked places instead of driving my car. I socialized and became involved in recreational pursuits. In other words, I got a *life*. It was truly exciting. The really cool thing was, I was still scarfing down a half-pint of ice cream every week as a reward for sticking to the program.

My third weigh-in confirmed that I was well on my way to hitting my goal. I'd lost another ten pounds, making a total weight loss over the three-month period of thirty-one pounds. I had gone from weighing 243 pounds to a rather svelte 212! Phenomenal, to say the least, especially for a guy who had all but given up on diets and exercise.

Truth of the matter was, this program I was following wasn't *really* a diet—not in the conventional sense, anyway. At least it didn't *feel* like one. That was really, really important to me.

Keep in mind that so much of the battle to lose weight is *in the mind*. Believing that this approach wasn't like a real diet—whether or not it really is doesn't enter into it—helped me conquer that vast wasteland of my mind. It was a slick trick that I learned as I developed it. It paid off in spades, given my results. Whether or not it's a diet is for the experts to sort out. I just know it worked.

There wasn't a flaw in the program that I could find in those initial three months. I ate well; I ate what I wanted; I ate when I wanted; and I always rewarded myself with that half-pint of ice cream each week that I stuck to it. I lost more than thirty pounds and trimmed more than five inches from my waist. I felt like I had enough energy to light a major metropolitan area. It was actually pretty painless and oh so easy.

I looked and felt great—this from a guy who abhors dieting and exercising. But like I said, it didn't *feel* like a diet, because I didn't have to give up any type of food. It all just sort of *happened*. If it happened for me, I just know it can happen for you as well.

I discovered that anything can happen if you set your mind to it and have faith that you're doing the right thing. I honestly believed that I could change my lifestyle, if only I could do it on my own terms and not be forced to do it all so quickly. When in my research I could not find a diet that suited me personally, I created a plan, not knowing for sure if it would be a success.

I mustered up all the faith I could garner and was determined to make it work—and work it did. I looked at my approach as a sort of St. Jude of weight loss—this was to be the last hope, the last attempt I would ever make at trying to lose weight. If I failed at this last-ditch effort, I would resign myself to forever remaining a fat person. I was prepared to sequester myself from people and simply retire from life. It could have been just that bad.

I customized this plan to require little effort on my part. It gave me what I had hoped for in all those other plans: a fighting chance to succeed. It encouraged me because at its core was a short-term approach. Trying to survive week to week was far more palatable than trying to survive over the course of, well, I didn't really know for how long.

That was the thing: I never knew when the end of the dieting would arrive. I knew there was no way I was going to diet for the rest of my life! This program even provided delectable rewards each week, short-term goals leading to long-term success. In other words, it was this fat man's dream plan.

CHAPTER EIGHT

THE GUERRILLA ATTACK

Remember the children's story about a princess who works up the courage to kiss a frog and transforms it into a handsome prince? That's how I felt three months after being on this plan. Like a prince, I mean. Okay, maybe not as handsome, but still the transformation was just as dramatic.

Where once a veritable recluse existed now lived a raving social butterfly. The seldom-chosen fat kid in the neighborhood now had an amazingly active social calendar, at least when compared to the number of previous social invitations. I was involved. I actually even dated on a semi-regular basis—though I must confess that I never really understood this social ritual very well. But that's a story for another time.

Surprise of surprises, I met someone of the fairer sex with whom I fell in love, eventually married, and started a family. My life was turning out grand!

That also turned out to be the beginning of a nightmare for me. It was at this allegedly blissful point in my life that an insidious guerrilla attack was launched. I didn't have a clue as to what was happening. But happen it did.

Oh, *Mea Culpa!*

One day as I got up from my easy chair, I realized that I could no longer see my feet for the size of my stomach. *Oh, God*, I thought, *I had become a person of profound poundage again! How could this have happened? Wasn't it just a short while ago that I had beaten the bulge? That I had dropped an enormous amount of weight? Hadn't I worked hard to keep it off? How could I let myself go to hell like this?* I was shocked and appalled as I gaped at my reflection in the mirror. There had been a sneak attack of fat, and it had taken me completely by surprise. Now it held me hostage.

I made a valuable discovery that day. I realized that being prone to weight gain is like being an alcoholic. The vice is different, of course, but we share a common state of mind. Just as the recovering alcoholic must guard against the temptation to drink alcohol, so too must people who love to eat to excess—like me—protect against the uncontrolled appetite. Otherwise, an average serving of food becomes a generous portion that then becomes two ... or three ... and pretty soon, the bulge has overtaken the midriff, the clothes are too danged tight, and you're standing in front of a full-length mirror, gaping at your reflection, scratching your balding head, and wondering: how *did* this happen? Was it even *possible* for the weight of the world to grab firmly onto my waist and I be none the wiser?

I learned that complacency is, without a doubt, a greater adversary than was the ritual of overeating. It is the greatest enemy that willpower-challenged people and others like us will ever face. Sure, there are support groups out there that you can join and lean on, but you must be *aware* that the problem exists—and be ready to *admit* that you have a problem—before you can become a groupie. Besides, it seems that a better way to solve the situation is to meet it squarely, face to face. Look it right in the eye, give it your best Clint Eastwood snarl, and make-its-day type of approach.

Actually, doing something yourself—especially when it is an extremely challenging task—does wonders in building self-esteem. As long as you *succeed*, that is.

That's how I solved the situation that confronted me in the mirror that day.

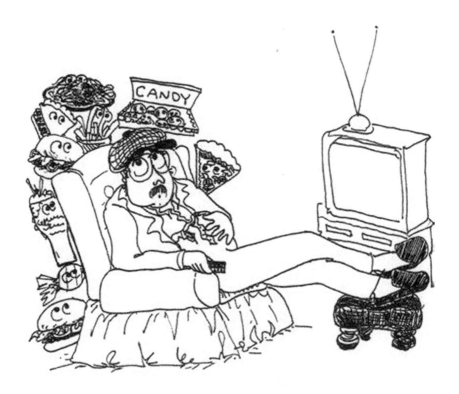

I realized that I could no longer see my feet for the size of my stomach.

The "Make My Day" Body Combat

After I got over the sight of my reflection, I got downright angry at myself—which, by the way, is one of only a half-dozen times that I've ever been angry—for being so stinking complacent that I would give in to the demon of delicious desires and those wonderful foods I loved to eat. I was mad—*fighting* mad—at myself. Mad that I'd reverted to that lazy lump of humanity from yesteryear. Mad that I hadn't seen it coming.

I really chewed myself out, but good, over the whole mess; then I set out to assess the damage.

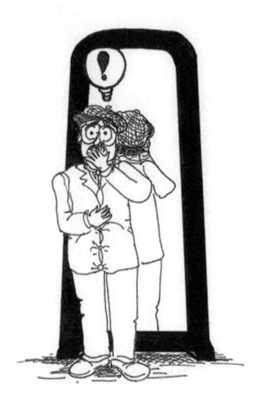

I was shocked as I gaped at my reflection in the mirror.

What I learned was shocking. I had jumped in weight to nearly 260 pounds, and my waist measured a "conservative" 45 inches. I was actually heavier at that precise juncture than at any other stage of my life. All because I just plain didn't care enough to keep on top of things.

So what did I do to make amends? I began by analyzing *what* and *when* I ate for an entire week. I visited my physician and went through a physical examination to confirm my suspicions. Does this sound vaguely familiar? It certainly should.

I set out on another campaign to beat the Battle of the Bulge, armed with the nuclear bomb of weight-loss programs that I had created for myself years ago.

Around every corner, tucked away in the dark recesses of every cabinet and cupboard, lurked the vile temptation of my enemy. I struggled with the bombardment of foodstuffs being lavished upon me. The twilight assaults and sniper attacks were constant, their force seemingly unrelenting. Yet I pressed forward, propelled by an overwhelming will to win and knowing that I could overcome any obstacle in my way—if I only kept focused on my reward at the end of the week.

But near the middle of that first week back on the approach, the pounding inside my stomach escalated to the force of a jackhammer on concrete. I wasn't sure how much more I could take.

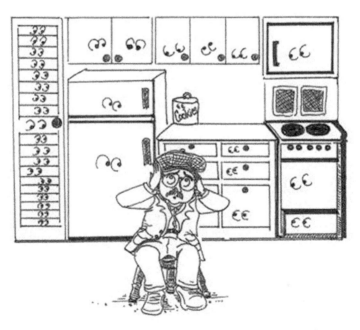

Tucked away in the dark recesses of every cabinet and
cupboard lurked the vile temptation of my enemy.

I was shell-shocked and weary from the constant battles. Honestly, I felt discouraged. My psyche—already fragile from this horrible quirk of fate that left me fatter than ever—was taking a beating. All those old taunts and jeers, the snide little asides being softly spoken about my weight gain, were murdering me. I wanted to give up and say *to hell with it.* But then, there was a light. A vision ...

CHAPTER NINE

ARMISTICE DAY

The light was the one that comes on when you open the refrigerator door. What made it so bright, I suppose, was that I had wandered into the kitchen in complete darkness and, with no other lights on, those things really shine pretty brightly.

You see, I had decided a few minutes earlier while tossing and turning in bed with those darned visions of sugarplums—among other stuff—dancing in my head, that I was going to raise the white flag of surrender and quit this weight-loss thing altogether.

I was obviously destined to be fat. Quite frankly, I didn't care at that point, as long as I could eat the leftover strawberry shortcake that was beckoning to me from the back of the refrigerator. *Que sera, sera.*

As I leaned into the confines of the old icebox and reached for my just desserts, something kind of spooky happened. An image appeared in my head. For a moment, I thought I was having one of those really weird religious experiences you often read about.

But on closer examination, I realized what it *really* was: my pot of gold at the end of the rainbow. I saw myself sitting on the steps of the local ice cream parlor, eating a half-pint of ice cream. The sun was shining brightly, warm on my face. There I was, smiling and looking quite content. And *thin.*

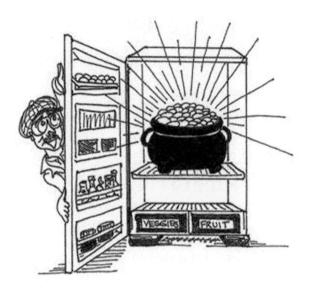

I thought I was having one of those really weird
religious experiences you often read about.

The whole image lasted all of maybe three or four seconds, certainly no longer than that. But it was just enough for me to close the door and go back upstairs to bed.

I knew at that very moment that I had not only fought the good fight, but I was going to come out on top—again. As I climbed those stairs that evening, I made a commitment to never become complacent again with regard to my eating and my lifestyle. I acknowledged that I was a person prone to porcine proportions, and would have to live with that for the rest of my life. I accepted it, unconditionally.

I practiced good old common sense and began modifying my eating. Over the next eight months of following the program, I lost seventy-five pounds and eleven inches from my waist. I had actually won the war. Not once, but *twice* ...

That last victory was nearly four decades ago. Today, I still practice this seemingly absurd approach because it's a way of life. It's pretty much second nature. Certainly, I continue to keep my guard up against the glancing blows of complacency, but I don't *consciously* do it. I've been following this approach for so many years now that I know when to say enough is enough. I have willpower. I've even treated myself to ice cream during the week on a number of occasions without backsliding into any nasty habits.

As this edition goes to press, my weight fluctuates between 185 and 190 pounds; my waist is 36 inches. As a matter of full disclosure, I should mention that in the original book, I had endured a bit better. I announced that my weight fluctuated between 174 and 178 pounds, and my waist size was 34 inches.

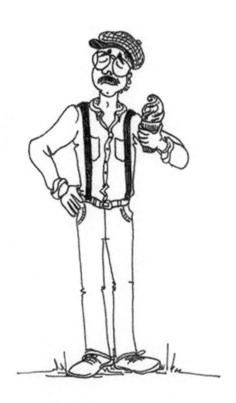

Ah! How sweet the taste of victory!

The difference can be attributed to two things. First, my weight is a bit more now than years ago because of certain medications I take—I consider that simply to be one of those vagaries of getting older.

Second—and perhaps more importantly—the slightly heavier weight that I carry now is the result of personal choice. I simply feel very good at my current weight.

The point is that I am in control these days. No longer do I sit in front of the television, feeding my face as my main source of exercise. Nowadays, my primary form of exercise is walking, with an occasional workout at a nearby fitness center. I take walks most mornings and often in the evening. When I drive somewhere, I often park my car farther away in parking lots, simply because I *enjoy* the walking. Why? Quite simply, I feel revitalized. I have energy to burn, and I just plain *feel* good.

CHAPTER TEN

PEACE-KEEPING EFFORTS
IN THE *WAIST* LAND

What I've discovered over the years of battling my weight problem is that there really is a light at the end of the proverbial tunnel. In the context of weight loss, however, that doesn't mean that people like you and me can take eating what we want when we want for granted.

To the contrary, it is incumbent upon us to be vigilant in our efforts to get and stay slimmer. It becomes imperative that we keep that vigilance acute once we get to the weight we want to be. Just as in military operations, it is often necessary to keep the peace in formerly hostile environments. So it is with our waistlines.

If you've followed this weight-loss approach through to the end—that is, you've reached what you have found to be your ideal weight—then the worst part of the war is over. You can celebrate your accomplishment without a bit of anxiety. That said, however, you need to ensure that you do not fall prey to an insurgency from all of those delectable dishes and tenacious temptations that seem to catch us off guard more often than not.

More than forty years have passed since I began my weight-loss journey. After seven-plus months, I'd lost all of the weight that I set out to lose. I was elated, to say the least. It was the first time I remember that I could actually see my feet when I stood up and looked down.

But it wasn't always easy to maintain the weight goals that I had achieved through my approach. I had to constantly monitor my actions—read, *watch my eating habits*—to ensure that I was keeping peace in my waistland. In doing that, I stopped just short of putting a few of those little plastic soldiers from my Battleground play set around my waist as a constant reminder to guard my waistland.

Fortunately, before I resorted to *that* particular tactic—and believe me, I probably would have if the plan I eventually came up with hadn't worked—I adopted a set of six tenets that helped me keep the excess weight off. Again, none of these is original. I picked them up from other diet plans and health-related reports that I had researched. The important consideration is that they work like a charm if you apply them to your life.

Tenet 1.

EAT ONLY IN THE ROOMS DESIGNED FOR THAT PURPOSE

This *is* the single most important tenet to live—and *eat*—by. It is absolutely imperative that you eat only in rooms that were designed for that purpose. You know, like the kitchen or the dining room, if you have one of the latter in your home as well. I'm pretty convinced that a greater number of pounds glommed onto my body as the result of eating while watching television in the living room and bedroom than from eating meals at the dinner table. Why? Because there is the tendency to become mesmerized by the drone of the television, which causes you to let your guard down instead of being vigilant and defending the waistland. Psychologically, people tend to eat a bit more mindlessly when "snacking." For example, it's really much easier, if not more fun, to eat chips straight from the bag from whence they came, rather than taking a moment or two to put a few in a *small*—that's the operative word here—bowl from which to munch. The same holds true for eating cookies—or anything else, for that matter. So, if you do no eating outside of those areas designed for that specific purpose, chances are you will successfully protect that waistland from the enemy. If you're still not convinced that it makes sense, go back and read chapter 8 again. If it happened to me, it could very well happen to you. In case you want to do it, don't extend the definition of "rooms designed for the purpose of eating" to include every room in which a television is located. Trust me, it happens. Pretty soon, you'll be eating snacks in bed. Just don't do it. Protect yourself against guerrilla attacks by not eating in front of *any* television, regardless of where it's located.

Tenet 2.
AVOID EATING WHEN YOU'RE NOT HUNGRY
This tenet is nearly as important as the first. What I discovered in my journey down the primrose path to weight loss was that I would catch myself eating just about anything that my chubby little hands could get ahold of, even though I wasn't the least bit hungry. No hunger pangs. No caving in to craving. Nothing. I just wanted to eat—maybe just to have something to do with the aforementioned chubby little hands. Then, of course, I had to sit down to savor every scrumptious bite, usually in front of the television. If you find yourself wanting to eat simply for the sake of eating, change whatever you're doing by working on a hobby instead. If you don't really have a hobby, find one. If you're like me and don't really have a hobby—other than eating, that is—simply go take a walk for a few minutes. The whole point is to change what you're doing and thinking at the time—your mind set and surroundings. It is a crucial change if you are to keep the peace on your waistland. If you begin doing other things at the moment you feel the urge to munch, it will eventually become a routine, and you'll be able to avoid eating when you're not hungry. It won't happen immediately,

but you will find it to be successful, if you give it a chance. *What if I'm hungry?* you might be asking about now. Well, that's where the next tenet comes in.

Tenet 3.
"GRAZE" THROUGHOUT THE DAY TO PLACATE YOUR HUNGER BETWEEN MEALS

For the most part, I've not bought into what the experts have to say concerning weight loss. But, alas, I must confess that they are spot-on with their recommendation that you "graze" throughout the day if you begin to get hungry between meals. I was actually astounded at how wonderfully this advice works. And strangely, it doesn't seem to be counterproductive, even if it *does* seem to be a bit counterintuitive. Let's say you finished that nice, healthy breakfast about an hour or an hour and a half ago and are now feeling a bit, shall we say, unfulfilled. Well, good for you! That means that you're making progress on your own personal journey to weight loss following this approach. Of course, that alone does nothing to placate those rumblings in your tummy. Instead of trying to fight them, however, go to the cupboard, grab a few whole-wheat crackers or even a couple of cookies and munch on them as you venture off to work on your hobby. It isn't much, but it works quite well in getting you to the next meal. I often rely on a banana to get me through. That said, usually for afternoon cravings, I grab three or four crackers and go about business as usual. Truth is, grazing throughout the day works. But a word of caution is necessary: don't graze with bowls of anything, even if it's healthy stuff. Eat fruit, like bananas or a handful of blueberries, if need be to get you through. You'll survive; I promise. One other word of caution: never, never eat anything that tastes nasty and bland (for me, this is a rice cake)— unless, of course, you like the taste of cardboard. Instead, try other things like celery and carrot sticks, which really are tasty too. The main thing to remember is that grazing is a stopgap measure to placate your hunger until the next meal. Grazing throughout the day also seems to leave you longing for less food at those regular meals. That is also a real plus. Any way you cut it, this is one of the best ways to protect your waistland against an insidious invasion from the enemy.

Tenet 4.
REMOVE STRESS FROM YOUR LIFE

Strange as it may seem, so many of our health problems can be linked directly to the amount of stress we allow into our lives. As research grows in this area, experts are finding that more and more illness can be attributable to what they call "bad" stress. Think about why you eat. At least in my case, if something didn't go particularly the way I wanted it to or thought it should, I'd make a beeline to the cupboard and grab as much food as I possibly could. Then I'd eat until my troubles were sent merrily on their way. I'm guessing this could be a reason why others eat as well. It stands to reason, by my way of thinking, that if you want to live a healthier life, you have to get rid of that nasty stress. That is often easier said than done, I know. Here's something else I learned about getting rid of stress—and this trumps just about anything else I *ever* learned: there are things in life over which you have control, and there are other things in life over which you have no control. The secret to living a nearly stress-free life is simple. Give those things in life over which you have no control to God—or your own personal spiritual power. I asked God to take on that task for me. It made all the difference in my life. That allowed me to deal only with those other nagging matters that I could control and dismiss quickly. As a result, my life is virtually stress-free, filled with joy and happiness, and extremely peaceful. If you follow this one simple—and yes, it really is simple—tenet, you will achieve all that you set out to accomplish. This I promise. It will also help you deal with the subject of the next tenet.

Tenet 5.

Don't Be Complacent

You've come this far, which is to say, you've finally developed that elusive concept called willpower and managed to knock off all the weight you set out to lose. What's next, you may ask? A good question. Before we get to that, you must prepare yourself for what could be the gravest enemy you'll ever face in the Battle of the Bulge: complacency. Of all the things that can undermine what you've attempted to accomplish, complacency is the worst. Many people who have lost a substantial amount of weight tend to become somewhat smug once it's all said and done. As I discovered—more than once or twice, I might add—weight has a way of creeping up on you and attaching itself to your waistline, without your even having a hint that it's happening. Do not let this happen to you! You have the power—and now, the energy—to keep that from occurring. All you have to do is keep in mind what your life was once like. Don't sit around and snack to your past levels. Instead, do something constructive. Do something to keep your mind sharp and focused at all times. Don't let the enemy sneak up on you without warning. How do you achieve that? There's one more piece of advice to follow, which reveals all.

Tenet 6.

Get Up, Get Out, and Do Fun Stuff

Now that you're well on your way to losing the weight you've always wanted to lose, now that your energy level has probably grown by leaps and bounds as a result of a slimmer you, it is time to take back your life! This simply means you should get up, get out, and enjoy this big, beautiful world of fun things to do. You are only restricted by your own imagination. Don't be afraid to show off the fruits of your weight-loss labor of love. If you're a bit hesitant, take tiny steps. Walk to the end of your driveway, smile, and wave at any neighbors you see. Then take a walk through your neighborhood. Step lively. Smile. Make it fun instead of a chore. Let your family, friends, and neighbors drink in your new look. You've not only chiseled out a new body, but you've got a whole new attitude to show off. Do it. As I mentioned earlier, my life changed dramatically— especially once I decided to get up and get out. I even eventually joined a fitness club. Interestingly, I woke up one morning to an absolutely beautiful day looming, and exclaimed to everyone within earshot that I was going to start jogging. What began as a silly, little urge became a routine. At one point, I was running about fifteen miles a week, just because I felt like it and because it was fun and surprisingly relaxing. Then, on many weekends, I participated in 5K runs being held throughout the area. I had a great time, and I wound up with a bunch of really cool T-shirts as a bonus! The thing is, I thoroughly enjoyed doing it and savored the camaraderie of the social aspect of the events. When I didn't feel like running, I got out and walked—if only to soak up the beauty of God's creation. If this sounds like a really tedious idea to you, walk with a purpose, like walking your dog. I'm telling you that life is so much better when you're out and about than when you're sitting inside doing whatever you're doing. Life is amazing! Get up, get out, and take it all in. There's a great big world out there just waiting for you to explore it. Besides, it will not only get your mind off eating, but it will keep you feeling good about yourself. Plain and simple.

Life is rich and full and vibrant. You no longer have any excuses for not participating in it. There are no secrets to living life to the hilt. All you have to do is make the effort.

I assure you that if you follow this approach to losing weight and make the effort to get out, you will discover a whole new world at your beck and call. You will be energized. You will want to do things that seemed impossible to attempt when you first began this journey. When you stop to consider how very simple anything in life can be, you'll realize that there are few—if any—doors that cannot be opened to you.

CONCLUSION

JUST DESSERTS

After years of attempting all kinds of diets, I realized that something had to change within the structure of those diets in order for me, a willpower-challenged person of enormous appetite, to lose the weight I needed to live a happy, healthy life.

It's certainly not an easy undertaking, but I was once told that anything worth having is worth working hard for. Mind you, I prefer an easier alternative, but there is a great deal of truth in that statement. I believe that the secret to getting something worthwhile is through working *smarter*, not harder.

In researching and writing this modest attempt at sharing my effort, I sought out the smarter way to lose weight—a way by which I could actually succeed. It involved pain and suffering. Well, actually it didn't—at least not *physically*. I just threw that in for effect. It did result in an awful lot of frustration, anguish, disappointment, and despair—and pretty much any other negative emotion or feeling known to mankind.

There came a point when I had to make a conscious decision regarding my future health. I could give up any further efforts to lose weight and simply resign myself to being one who is obnoxiously obese for the rest of my life. On the other hand, I could reach deep inside—do a gut check, as it were—and find a solution to my problem through a better way. I chose to take it upon myself to lose weight. But that's only part of this story. As you read through this approach, you may have picked up on an undercurrent of *psychological* warfare as well as the obvious attacks discussed. This is crucial, not only to this approach but to living life to its fullest. Without the right attitude, you are only going to sell yourself short and, quite possibly, fail to achieve all that you can in life.

One statement to remember, above all else, is this: *you are only limited by your personal perceptions of your limitations.* The truth is, you can—and *will*—accomplish anything you put your mind to achieving. The problem most people have is that they set their sights on doing something that they perceive as being beyond their level of belief in themselves, and manage to talk themselves out of attempting it— oftentimes before they hardly begin. The truth is, you have to believe in your dream.

The Brazilian writer Paulo Coelho, in the introduction to his seminal novel, *The Alchemist*, cited four obstacles that often prevent a person from garnering the courage to confront their dream.

After reading this novel, I honestly believed that I could accomplish anything I set my mind on achieving simply by understanding that one little concept: *I am only limited by my own perceptions of my limitations.* This, I believe, is the essence of overcoming Coelho's four obstacles. This revelation literally changed my outlook on life.

The day I began my weight-loss saga was the first day of my life that I actually believed I was taking control. I decided I was no longer going to let negativity influence my life in *any* way.

Where I once became discouraged by things happening or not happening in my life, I began taking every negative that occurred and dissecting it until I found a positive to trump the negative. That's the key: finding a positive within a negative and running with it. The positive is there, trust me. I don't care what the negative is—and believe me, I've had more negatives occur in my life than I care to think about, let alone count. But in each instance, I flipped it into a positive and I thrived.

My point is simple: if you truly believe you can achieve something—whether it's as innocuous as a small routine task or huge like losing weight by some unconventional approach—you will accomplish it. You just have to believe in yourself. This cannot be overstated. Always believe that there is nothing beyond your reach.

Believe in yourself and what you're doing at any given time, and good things will fall into your lap—a lap that is far less ample than it was before, if you followed my approach, I might add. You have to want something bad enough to convince yourself that you can accomplish it. That's how you wind up believing in yourself. That's how you no longer become limited by your own perceptions of your limitations. It works. I am living proof.

There's nothing else to tell and only one thing left for you to do: get with it. I mentioned this early on, but it merits repeating. I obviously cannot guarantee that my weight-loss program will work for you. All I can say is that it has worked for me—not once, but *twice*—when no other weight-reduction plan did. Other times, when I caught myself slipping, the approach was there to get me back on track. While I may have failed *it*, my method never let me down. Never, ever.

This plan worked because it was designed specifically with the anti-diet, anti-exercise freak in mind. Me. There are no tricks, no gimmicks, and absolutely no sacrifices. This program is really nothing more than good old common sense and intuition with a healthy dose of positive reinforcement. Maybe with a pinch of positive attitude thrown in. That's it.

While guarantees cannot be made, remember that there's a good chance we share many of the same qualities. I had tried many diet programs—both the conventional and the unorthodox. I spent beaucoup bucks trying to get rid of my ever-expanding waistline without success. Why? Because every diet I ever attempted wanted me to work hard at losing weight, and honestly, I just didn't want to. My family doctor reinforced the notion that I shouldn't *have* to work hard to lose weight. Besides, I was essentially lazy and didn't have an abundance of willpower. Who am I kidding? I had absolutely *no* willpower!

What I discovered was that I do have an abundance of common sense. By capitalizing on that strength, I managed to overcome a lot of glaring weaknesses, like eating too much and exercising all too infrequently. The approach worked for me. All you have to do is believe!

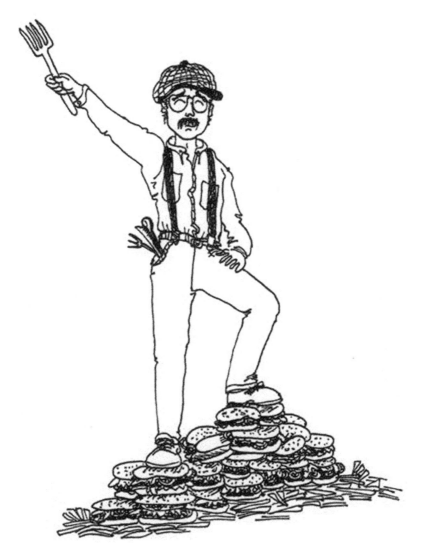

You really are only limited by your personal
perceptions of your limitations. Believe!

ABOUT THE AUTHOR

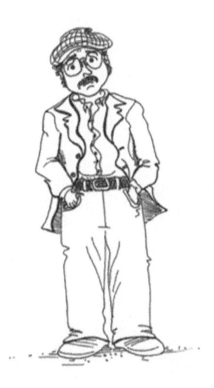

Thom Slagle never could make up his mind as to what he actually wanted to be when he finally grew up. He tried several occupations, none of which really interested or amused him, before settling on life as a writer.

He resides in Florida.

HELPINGS

Quick Reference Guide

After you've completed my weight-loss program, there may be times when you may want to refer to specific pointers that are core elements of the plan. This section provides a quick reference to guide you to the attack plans outlined, and the tips and tenets that appear in the text.

The Attack Plans

Tips to Get You through the Struggles

The Six Tenets

Daily Analysis Sheet

Included in this section of the book is one Daily Analysis Sheet that you may copy and use to log your food consumption as you set your personal agenda to begin your weight-loss journey. If you choose to create your own forms, make sure you include all of the vital section headers.

DAILY ANALYSIS SHEET

WEEK		DATES		DAY	
MEAL	WHAT I ATE			AMT	TIME OF DAY

Key: B = Breakfast L = Lunch D = Dinner S = Snack

Milton Keynes UK
Ingram Content Group UK Ltd.
UKHW011825061123
432058UK00003B/69